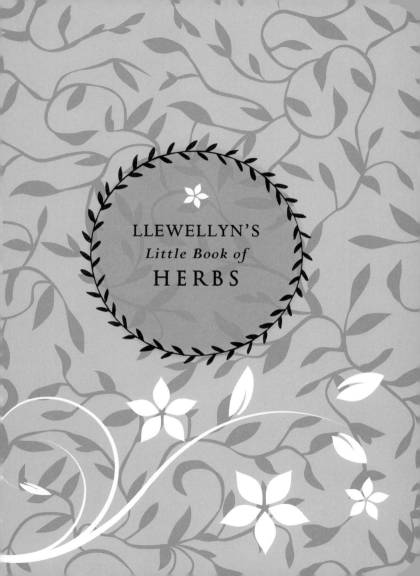

LLEWELLYN'S
Little Book of
HERBS

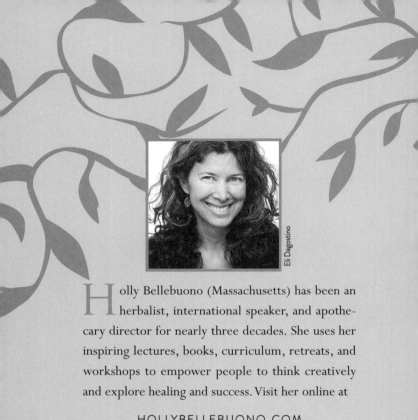

Eli Dagostino

Holly Bellebuono (Massachusetts) has been an herbalist, international speaker, and apothecary director for nearly three decades. She uses her inspiring lectures, books, curriculum, retreats, and workshops to empower people to think creatively and explore healing and success. Visit her online at

HOLLYBELLEBUONO.COM

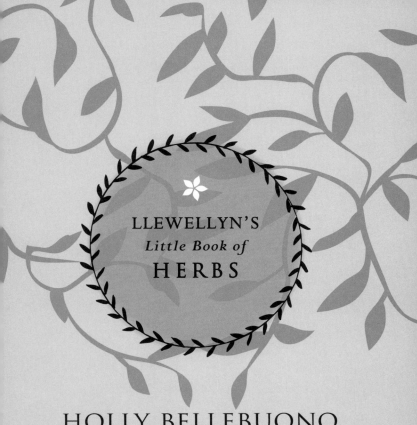

LLEWELLYN'S
Little Book of
HERBS

HOLLY BELLEBUONO

LLEWELLYN PUBLICATIONS
WOODBURY, MINNESOTA

FIRST EDITION
Second Printing, 2021

Book design by Rebecca Zins
Cover cartouche by Freepik
Cover design by Lisa Novak and Shira Atakpu

Llewellyn Publications is a registered trademark of Llewellyn Worldwide Ltd.

Library of Congress Cataloging-in-Publication Data
Names: Bellebuono, Holly, author.
Title: Llewellyn's little book of herbs / Holly Bellebuono.
Other titles: Little book of herbs
Description: Woodbury, Minnesota : Llewellyn Worldwide, Ltd, 2020. |
Series: Llewellyn's little book series; 12
Identifiers: LCCN 2019053979 (print) | LCCN 2019053980 (ebook) | ISBN 9780738762050 (print) | ISBN 9780738762784 (ebook)
Subjects: LCSH: Herbals. | Medicinal plants. | Herb gardening. | Herbs—Therapeutic use.
Classification: LCC RM666.H33 B4574 2020 (print) | LCC RM666.H33 (ebook) | DDC 615.3/21—dc23
LC record available at https://lccn.loc.gov/2019053979
LC ebook record available at https://lccn.loc.gov/2019053980

Llewellyn Worldwide Ltd. does not participate in, endorse, or have any authority or responsibility concerning private business transactions between our authors and the public.

All mail addressed to the author is forwarded, but the publisher cannot, unless specifically instructed by the author, give out an address or phone number.

Any internet references contained in this work are current at publication time, but the publisher cannot guarantee that a specific location will continue to be maintained. Please refer to the publisher's website for links to authors' websites and other sources.

Llewellyn Publications
A Division of Llewellyn Worldwide Ltd.
2143 Woodale Drive
Woodbury, MN 55125-2989
www.llewellyn.com

Printed in China

The recipes, suggestions, and ideas in this book are based on the author's personal experience and are not meant to constitute medical advice. For illnesses, consult a health care professional.

ACKNOWLEDGMENTS

Warm thanks to my friends with whom I've enjoyed gardens and flowers for years: Laurisa, Zoe, Lisa, Kristina, Tarah, and Missy; and to the students with whom I've delighted in sharing herb stories and adventures: Ellen, Keya, Sasha, Patty, Janice, and many more who have graced my gardens with their presence and enthusiasm. Gratitude to my wonderful sister, Leslie, for always being there for me. Much love to my children, Gabriel and Madia; I'm so proud of you both! May your life experiences be creative and meaningful. Deep love and thanks to my dear David, my loving partner; your support for my work makes me smile, and our friendship means the world to me.

Thanks to my agent, Jody Kahn, and to the people at Llewellyn, who help empower us all one book at a time.

Contents

Exercises

Tips

Charts

INTRODUCTION

Greetings! Welcome to the world of growing and using medicinal herbs. Whether you are a seasoned gardener and you want to put all those abundant plants to use or you've made salves and oils before but never tried growing your own herbs—or any number of other plant/craft combinations—this book is for you. You may be eyeing your garden space right now, imagining where to plant the basil, or you may be hunkered down in a snowstorm perusing seed catalogs. Perhaps you're sitting on a small porch or balcony and dreaming about beautiful herbs growing in pots. Maybe you've just sampled a little jar of beeswax salve and you're wondering how to make something similar yourself. Wherever you are, and whatever your background with plants is, know that this book is a friendly welcome from an herbalist who has spent years learning, experimenting, and enjoying growing herbs and using their wonderful medicines—and it will help you do the same.

Herbs are a welcoming enterprise. Working with plants is a lovely way to spend your time, and not only is it therapeutic and enjoyable, it's also functional because we can make so many helpful and healing remedies with plants. It can boost confidence to know that you can be in charge of your own health, using plants as both foods and medicines to support a healthy lifestyle. Many men and women enjoy the ability to support their families and communities through simple remedies for common health issues, such as cough, runny nose, indigestion, and difficulty sleeping. Not only is it cost-effective to grow and use your own herbs, but it is heartening to know that you can provide for your family. It is also exciting to learn more about a heritage and tradition that has been a cornerstone of many lives for centuries.

A Bit About Me

When I was a kid, I was a Nature kid, with a capital N. Though I grew up in the suburbs of Asheville, our little valley was surrounded by the Blue Ridge Mountains and was secluded enough that the road through the valley was a dead-end road, and the narrow strip of 1950s houses along the road backed onto sprawling fields, rugged cow pastures, and mountain slopes that ascended all the way to the Blue Ridge Parkway. I loved being outside and would spend hours playing in our backyard, creating rock forts in the little creek that ran behind our house and building structures in the treehouse my dad had built for my brother and sister and me. I scooped up the inch-long crawdads in the creek, I went on long walks to pet the horses in the nearby field, and I sucked the ends off honeysuckle flowers for the sweet flavor. In high school I longed to join 4-H and garden, but my parents had more "civilized" plans for me and I instead focused on creative writing, which I loved.

I ended up working in Atlanta at a publishing house, as an assistant editor for several magazines or trade journals on, of all things, aircraft. But it didn't last long—my heart was calling for me to get back into nature and experience it more deeply, so I moved back to the mountains of North Carolina—a little further north from Asheville, where I grew up—and settled in Boone, getting my master's degree at Appalachian State. Here I literally dove into outdoor programs by spelunking with the caving program and immersing myself in dark, curvy caves with dripping sounds and swooshing bats and cold, wet rocks, whitewater rafting on the Nolichucky and Nantahala Rivers, and experimenting with gardening. Working with plants nurtured my deep understanding of energy, feminine consciousness, and the spiritual connectedness of all things. I quickly found myself on the fulfilling journey of plant spirit medicine and herbal healing.

The Joy of Making Herbal Remedies for Yourself and Your Family

If you're creating medicines for yourself or your family, this book provides helpful ideas to keep you safe, to give you creative license, and to get children on board with natural healing.

Being a home herbalist is rewarding for so many reasons: it is a sustainable, economical way to keep yourself and your family healthy. Because you can harvest your own medicines, you need not rely on a pharmacy or doctor for the most common illnesses we all deal with. It's also a very enjoyable education in many aspects of life: botany, biology, climate, soil sciences, chemistry, horticulture, anatomy, and physiology. The combination of this learning is enriching and will last a lifetime.

Working with herbs is one of the most fulfilling ways to spend your time, and it's also quite easy. Don't be intimidated by Latin names or feeling that it might not be safe; on the contrary, this book will focus on the many very safe herbs to grow, harvest, and use. Rest assured that the herbs in this book are excellent and safe choices with which you can experiment and gain knowledge.

Working with herbs can also be lively! Consider joining classes, workshops, online courses, or apprenticing with someone who already has years of experience with plants. This will skyrocket your understanding—and therefore your enjoyment—of herbalism. Hands-on classes, especially, will promote your ability and skill in preparing herbal remedies and cosmetics, keeping you healthy and comfortable. Check your local area for herbalists who teach classes, go online, and allow yourself the luxury of traveling every so often to reach events and conferences outside your region. It will be worth it not only for the information on plants but also the networking and mingling that is so wonderful with a group of people who share plants in common.

Also, don't underestimate the things you can do as a home herbalist: you can invest in your own health, catalogue the plants on your property and around you, and pique your children's interest in Mother Nature. You can also stock your own medicine pantry with remedies that will be needed at various times of the year by making fire cider with spicy herbs and vinegar, tinctures with antiviral herbs, and first aid ointments to soothe everything from scratches to burns.

Finally, you may become so enamored with making herbal remedies that you become a teacher yourself, sharing your knowledge with others and making a difference in your community. Let this practical little book guide you in learning practical methods of gardening and crafting medicines. Remember to let yours and the plants' inner voices shine through, and give yourself time to sit, reflect, and listen.

How to Use This Book

This book is arranged in a way that follows what will likely be the hands-on cycle you experience with plants. First, in chapter 1 you'll learn about growing the herbs—getting your hands in the dirt and experiencing what is, for many, a very therapeutic feeling. One of the cornerstones of this book is the herb lists; I'll provide you with several lists of herbs in various categories to help you decide which plants you want to work with. These will be the herbs on which we focus throughout the whole book. Chapter 1 explores easy and useful herbs for you to consider starting out with because they are very safe, or because they're incredibly easy to grow, or because they make simple healing remedies.

Additionally, this chapter provides unusual or "next-level" herbs, which are also safe and easy and will provide you with more options for making medicines. Some of these plants require a warm climate or a greenhouse or cold frame, though most can be grown in nearly any climate; these will give you an opportunity to expand your experience with both growing and crafting. A third list in this chapter details useful herbs that grow wild, and it shares how to identify, harvest, and use them. The last list gives examples of herbs that are best not planted in gardens or even in pots because they can run rampant and take over. We will also explore creative ways and places to grow herbs, as well as things to consider when you're growing herbs, such as a plant's height, its soil requirements, and how annuals, biennials, and perennials fit in your plan.

Chapter 2 explores various methods of harvesting these plants. You'll learn about using the lunar cycle and how to harvest throughout the seasons. We will cover the easiest and best ways to harvest all parts of the plant—the flowers, seeds, leaves, and roots—and you'll get tips for drying your herbs or using them fresh.

Chapter 3 explores various creative methods of crafting with the plants and making functional medicines, cosmetics, and items that bring joy. You'll learn how to make teas, beeswax salves, lotions, spritzers, infused honeys, vinegars, and more. This chapter is full of exercises and recipes for simple remedies using the plants on these lists, so you can grow comfortable with these handfuls of plants and discover how versatile they are, using them again and again in different ways.

Finally, chapter 4 provides guidance on using the medicines, storing them, and using basic recipes in creative ways. You'll find ways to take the foundations you made in chapter 3 and apply them in additional remedies and recipes. You'll also get tips for organizing baskets of your premade goodies to give as gifts.

As you go through this book, remember to allow for beauty in your garden. It may seem obvious, but sometimes we forget that our food and herb production facility is really a garden that is innately and inherently lovely. Indulge in fun things like bird feeders, wind chimes, glass gazing balls, statuary, and artwork. Also remember to notice the little things, to appreciate the small parcels of beauty that are gifted to us almost every moment:

- the songs of birds
- the feel of dry, soft earth sifting through your fingers
- the glint of water droplets on a leaf
- your cat, who pushes against your leg while you're weeding
- the red of the tractor, the yellow of the flower, the brown of the wood

- how the warm sun feels on your neck and shoulders
- the acrid or sweet smell of the roots you pull up
- how a dozen honeybees can fit on a large flower head, tipping it sideways
- the bitter or minty taste of a medicinal herb on the tongue
- how your empty lightweight bag is suddenly heavy with your harvest

Enjoy all this beauty and let it fill you up. Savor these moments, as they are just as healing as any dosage from a tincture bottle.

Let's get started with herbs! We will dive into the garden, that luscious vehicle of wonder and greenness that will blossom into our herbal apothecary, filling our shelves with remedies and our hearts and bodies with health, wellness, and wholeness.

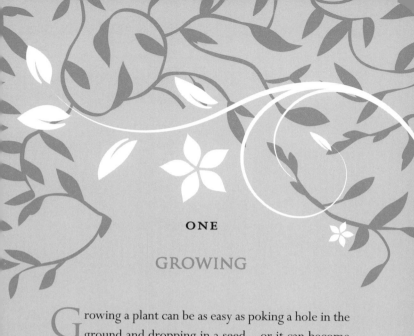

ONE

GROWING

G rowing a plant can be as easy as poking a hole in the ground and dropping in a seed—or it can become a complex endeavor that involves seed-sourcing catalogs, garden design and planning, plumbing and irrigation, site development, permaculture methods, the introduction of pollinators, and even getting town, county, or housing association permission. Let's assume you are a plant lover who is ready to grow edible and medicinal herbs to support your health. There are a variety of places to grow plants and many ways to go about it.

Planning Your Growing Space

Certain environmental considerations will help you decide what kind of herbs to grow and where to grow them. For instance, some herbs prefer sun or shade, some require a certain type of soil, some have height considerations, and some are short-lived, while others, once planted, may be part of your life for years. Consider the following options when thinking about which herbs to grow.

Where to Grow

Growing and using medicinal herbs is for everyone— regardless whether you have acres to farm, a small yard, or a simple balcony or windowsill.

A garden for medicinal herbs need not be large; many people grow a small garden of ten-by-ten feet. This is plenty of space to grow a number of helpful herbs that you can harvest and turn into medicines. For instance, in this small space you could grow several lemon balms, a catnip, two or three valerian, a nice large yarrow, some lavender, and several calendulas, and still have room to walk between them. A small garden plot is a great way to experiment without investing in big tools such as plows or tillers; all you'll need is a shovel and a rake.

If you don't have garden space or don't want to create a garden plot, you can still enjoy growing edible and medicinal plants in pots. Many plants grow well in pots, especially the Mediterranean plants such as sage, rosemary, and fennel, and others such as anise hyssop and catnip. Plastic pots are good at keeping the soil evenly moist; if you choose terra-cotta pots, place some moss, mulch, or wood chips on top of the soil to help keep the water from evaporating.

Gardening with pots is convenient in many ways: the pots can be moved, the pots can serve as a hedge or boundary, and they make experimenting easy. Be sure to move pots from indoors to outdoors carefully so that you don't shock a plant, keeping in mind that the temperature difference can be substantial. Move indoor plants or seedlings outside during the day for a few hours and return the pot indoors at night, at least until the plant gets accustomed to the new temperatures.

Another option for growing plants is to join a community garden, where you can rent or share space. These plots often have access to tillers and watering hoses, and the entire garden is often already fenced in. Many community gardens have CSA programs, or community supported agriculture, where you can sign up to purchase vegetables and herbs grown by others in your shared space. Be aware that they might have rules against growing self-seeding herbs such as stinging nettle or root-traveling herbs such as mugwort, which can take over a garden patch.

Finally, if you have a lawn, some seeds can be sprinkled along the edge of the lawn, especially near a fence or border. This is a neat way to get edible and medicinal plants for the picking without lifting a shovel or creating a garden, which may not be permitted in some neighborhoods. Sprinkle seeds in the fall or early spring where the grass is thin but there is good sun exposure; good choices are calendula and fennel seeds. These are annuals that will sprout for one season only and can be harvested and put to use. Seeds are best gleaned from a friend's plants, but if you're purchasing seeds, look for non-GMO seeds and those grown from organically raised plants. Residue from chemicals sprayed onto plants to kill pests or weeds will be in their seeds and can compromise the viability and safety of the new plant.

Tucking Herbs Elsewhere

Part of the joy of gardening is getting unexpected herbs from friends or finding lovely little plants at a market and adding them to your garden. It's easy to do with medicinal herbs, too. Tuck rosemary against a south-facing wall where it can soak up the sun and be protected from winter winds; tuck violets anywhere it's wet and damp and shady. Plant St. John's wort or yarrow on earthen mounds that have been formed from excavation or landscaping; tuck mints along the edges of the garden, and plant gifts of lemon balm, self-heal, or holy basil in the sunny spots near your driveway or back door.

Sun or Shade?

Certain herbs require shade and others prefer sun. Thankfully, many will tolerate a combination and flourish wherever you put them. Lemon balm will grow fine in the sun but grows happily in the shade with broad dark green leaves that are succulent and juicy. Yarrow, sage, and pleurisy root all prefer full sun, while catnip is happy in partial shade. Elderberry, a large shrub, likes to keep her feet wet, so planting her somewhere swampy or marshy is best (perhaps under the eaves of the house or near a drain). Mints are surprising; they will grow almost anywhere, from lush meadows to roadside wastelands. Spearmint and peppermint are quite happy in full sun, but I've also been surprised to come across mints growing in the middle of a stream, completely in the water, where they were thriving. Similarly, jewelweed wants to be very wet, so if you have access to damp woodlands or a creek, consider planting jewelweed.

When you're planting a garden or arranging pots with herbs, think about where the sun hits the land. The side of the house that gets morning sun will be good for delicate herbs that prefer shade; this is because the other side of the house—the side that gets afternoon sun—usually experiences the sun for longer and the heat is often more intense. Plant Mediterranean herbs such as sage, lavender, and rosemary on the side with the most sun. If you're working with potted plants, elevate them on a deck for better light or tuck them under shrubs or trees to cool them off and provide shade.

Thinking About Soil

Without getting into the elements and minerals that make soil what it is—such as phosphorus, nitrogen, and potassium—let's think about types of soil. Is it cakey or sandy? Does it hold water or does water drain well? Clay generally holds water and needs to be broken up with sand, grit, compost, or loam. Sand is too porous and needs clay and soil added to it.

To test what sort of soil you have, simply squeeze a handful in your fist. If it all sticks together, it likely needs to be more porous. If it crumbles and is too dry, it needs more loam or clay. It's easy to remedy this for a small garden plot or pots simply by combining what you need in a wheelbarrow with a small shovel.

When you're filling a pot, place gravel or stones on the bottom to encourage proper water drainage. Make sure the soil will stay damp but not too wet. Also select a pot that is slightly larger than necessary; plants grow quickly, and this will keep you from having to repot too frequently. It will also ensure the plant does not become root-bound.

If you live in an area with lots of oak trees, your soil is likely acidic. Amend it with materials that make it more alkaline, such as manure or compost. If you live near the coast, your soil may be sandy; be sure to enrich it with compost or loam. A quick visit to a garden center will help you determine your soil needs. Purchase small bags of what you need, and don't forget that adding compost from your kitchen, leaves, and other organic materials can be helpful.

Plant Height

It may be helpful to consider a plant's height when you're deciding what to grow. In my herb garden, I created three large beds starting at our deck and heading outward. The plants in the bed closest to the deck are generally short plants, growing at a height of no more than one to two feet: I planted short fennel, lemon balm, oregano, and sage. The second bed contains herbs that grow about four feet tall: bee balm, anise hyssop, yarrow, and pleurisy root. In the third bed, the plants are quite tall: these include vitex, elderberry, and valerian. It's worked quite well and has a great visual appeal.

Depending on your region and climate, certain herbs will grow to different heights, and you can use this to your advantage. Thyme is often grown as a ground cover, meaning it literally can be walked upon, and many people do this because it releases a lovely scent. Other herbs are low growing; garlic, for instance, is a very short plant, barely reaching knee height when it flowers. This, along with calendula and lavender, can be placed in a small bed, hedge, or pot. Valerian and elecampane, on the other hand, are towering herbs that grow much taller than most people. These are best placed against a fence or by a gate, or a long a border where they can be staked.

Annuals, Biennials, and Perennials

Not all herbs will grow forever. Think about whether you will plant herbs that come and go in one year (annuals) or herbs that may be around for decades (perennials). Plants come in several types, most notably annuals, biennials, and perennials.

ANNUALS (in my time zone; yours may be different) include fennel, dill, calendula, and basil. Catnip is usually an annual and it self-seeds freely, as do portulaca, wild geranium, and tansy. St. John's wort behaves as a biennial (though it is botanically a perennial and in warmer

climates it reliably returns year after year) and wild yarrow does too, though cultivated yarrow is a perennial.
Almost all vegetables are annuals, though many kales and
cabbages will return the following spring. Herbs that are
perennials in tropical climates, such as turmeric, will
only hang around for one winter where I live in Massachusetts and must be treated as an annual. This means
the plant is dug up and harvested (for the root) and you
must replant the following year, either from seeds or a
seedling. Rosemary is another herb that prefers warmth
in order to behave as a perennial; otherwise it's an annual.
I've had winters where rosemary lives and winters where
rosemary dies.

BIENNIALS are plants that generally have a two-year
lifespan. Usually they will sprout in their first year and
grow short or low to the ground, producing only leaves
or a rosette low against the soil. In their second year, they
will send up a stalk with flowers that will go to seed.
Where I live, elecampane and valerian are biennial, as is
Queen Anne's lace. When you find the basal rosette of
a biennial, leave it where it is or transplant it, knowing
that it will send up its stalk the following year to produce flowers and seeds. For instance, I do this frequently
with motherwort, a biennial I welcome everywhere I find

her. When this useful herb shows its pointy little leaves, I carefully transplant it where I want it to grow, knowing it will reach its fullest potential later that year or the following year. It can grow quite tall and shrubby—reaching shoulder height and growing full—so be sure to give it plenty of space.

PERENNIALS are plants that return again and again, often having quite a long lifespan of many years. They reliably come back every spring, making them an easy cornerstone of your garden. You can plan your garden around perennials such as sage, oregano, and roses. Stinging nettles are perennials and they also self-seed rampantly, so think carefully about where you want your nettle patch! Within twenty yards of your planting, you will find new nettles growing wild.

Elderberry bushes are perennial; I have a wonderful elderberry patch near me. They are larger than bushes, more like trees, so they're not a good option to plant in a pot. I need a ladder to reach them, or I'll drive a pickup truck up to them to reach the tops. Plant elderberries where they can keep their feet wet and their heads in the sun; along a creek or next to a drain is a good location. Sage is also perennial, though where I live it tends to flower for a few years and then starts to get spindly and sparse. It will continue to live for years, but its gray-green leaves will never be as fat, round, and lush as they were its first couple of years, though they will always be astringent, antimicrobial, and useful.

Many perennial herbs like to be cleaved after a few years, meaning you can dig up a portion of them and transplant it elsewhere. Oregano, for instance, grows wider and wider, forming a mat. It's easy to take a sharp digging spade and cut squares from the main plant. For instance, from an oregano mat that is approximately three-by-three feet, I will dig out two or three eight-inch-square sections. Take your spade and push it straight down with a quick, sharp movement, making a clean slice through the plant and its roots. Pull up your square and plant it elsewhere, keeping the top level with the soil where you've moved it and pressing down (I use the heel of my boot) to press out any air from around the roots. You want it to fit tightly in its new hole. Water immediately and soon you'll have a new oregano mat. Other herbs I've cleaved include cultivated yarrow, bee balm, lavender, and any plant that is grown as a ground cover that forms a mat.

All of these elements (sun/shade, type of soil, height, and whether it is an annual, biennial, or perennial) will help you decide what herbs you'd like to try growing first. If in doubt, plant it; it's better to learn by trial and error than not try at all.

Creating a Home for Your Herbs

Whether you grow your herbs in a garden or in pots, these tips will help you keep your plants healthy and increase your enjoyment of the growing process.

Mulch

Mulch in the garden is a priority, both for the health of the plants and your own comfort. Mulch the pathways for walking and the beds to keep down weeds. There are a variety of mulches to choose from: grass clippings from a lawn mower work well, as does straw (but not hay, which is full of seeds). Where I live near the coast, people use seagrass, a type of seaweed.

Wood chips also work, but because wood chips don't entirely cover the ground, sprouts can poke through, so it's a good idea to purchase a cloth ground cover and lay down two layers in the walking paths, spreading the mulch over the top. Replace the ground cover in three to four years, and replace the mulch regularly too.

TIP 2

Moving Herbs Inside

Some herbs are sensitive to cold and must be moved indoors in the winter. These include rosemary, which is also sensitive to dry air, so keep the indoor humidity high enough. If it dries out, it will drop its needles and wither. Move plants to a bay window where they get natural light, and then screen off the window with plastic wrap so the air around them stays fairly moist. Don't place plastic wrap directly on the top of the soil in the pot, as this causes mold to grow; instead, keep the entire plant moist by creating a mini greenhouse. Introduce the plant back outside in the spring carefully, taking it out only for a few hours at a time for a week or so to avoid shock.

Fences and Boundaries

If you live where deer roam freely or near pastures with cows or goats that can escape, you'll recognize the value of a strong, high fence. In my early days, I tapped light little poles into the ground and affixed three-foot-high fencing with the little twist ties that you wrap around a loaf of bread. Needless to say, the fences fell, the poles leaned over, and the veggies and herbs I had so tenderly tended were munched happily by the local deer population. Borrow a friend's post-hole digger and invest some time in creating a strong backbone for your fence, and install six-foot-high fencing. An alternative to a fence is to create your garden next to a wall of the house and use potted plants as boundaries on the other sides. Potted plants will keep dogs out and expand the amount of room you have to grow, creating a beautiful boundary.

Watering Your Herbs

If you can, install a sprinkler or watering system for water-loving herbs such as elderberry, nettle, mallow, and black cohosh. (A sprinkler will also be helpful for vegetables.) Find hoses and a sprinkler that suits you, and position them so that they water what you need watered. Also make sure the on/off switch is easy to access, preferably at the house so you don't have to enter a wet garden to turn it off. If a sprinkler system is not an option, keep a hose and a watering can handy.

 Cover the watering can with a tarp or store it in a shed to keep it free of leaves and debris that can clog the shower head.

Chairs and Benches

It's lovely to sit in the middle of a sweet little garden and just enjoy it. A small bench or chair also can be a welcome relief after bending or kneeling, and it invites someone else to spend time with you while you weed. An easy way to create a bench is to take a small plank of wood and position it in a corner of a raised bed or between two beds to make a quick low seat. You can also place two small chairs with a little table between them somewhere in the garden. Why not sip your rose petal, lemon balm, or anise hyssop iced tea while you're sitting next to your roses, lemon balm, and anise hyssop? There's something charming about creating a living space for people within a living space for plants.

Raised Beds or Regular Beds

A raised bed is a plot of land that has been dug and prepared and then contained by building a small wall around it. Often the wall is made of four simple planks of wood that create a box. A regular bed is a prepared bed without the box. There are pros and cons to raised beds and regular beds; I've done it both ways and enjoy them both.

RAISED BEDS offer clear delineations about what's growing where. They add an element of organization to what could otherwise be a wild and rampant garden (which is what most of my gardens end up becoming), and they give a sense of order that is nice, especially in the early part of the season when you are putting seeds and seedlings out.

Raised beds can be higher than the ground around them by a foot or more. Raised beds, though, can be *too* big—their width can seem reasonable at first, but later they feel too wide, and you discover you can't comfortably reach halfway across. I've also found that because raised beds can be filled with more soil, I am tempted to plant more plants in them, but at the end of the summer I face a jungle of plants that seem overburdened and are spilling out into the paths, creating obstacles. And when the raised bed boards begin to rot after a few years, they'll need replacing.

REGULAR BEDS are great, too: they offer ease of access and can be as narrow or as wide as you want, though the pathways can merge with the beds and lose their boundaries.

> I recommend building a narrow bed up against the inside of your fence and using the fence as the boundary, rather than having a walking path along the inside of the fence. Be vigilant about weeding the exterior of the fence (outside the garden). This is a great use of space, and the fence doubles as a structure upon which you can grow climbing vines such as hops, cucumbers, gourds, and beans.

Whichever type of bed you choose, be sure to allow plenty of room to walk between them.

Greenhouses and Cold Frames

If you'd like to grow herbs from seed, you might have good luck doing it in a greenhouse or a cold frame. Greenhouses have a way of capturing our imaginations, inviting us to dwell in a space of warmth and sun; much like a cathedral, they guide our gaze upward at the ceiling. Greenhouses are magical spaces in the depths of winter, cushioning orchids or rare flowers or lime and lemon trees, warming trays of seeds, or even just serving as a calm place out of the weather to store coiled-up hoses and trowels.

GREENHOUSES are magnificent. I grew up in Asheville, North Carolina, and often visited the Biltmore Estate, where I would wander dreamily through the incredible greenhouses that were built there in the early 1900s with their wrought-iron frames housing two-story-tall palm trees. Quirky hippie greenhouses that are cobbled and patched together out of random building supplies also look whole, intact, and inviting. Some people hang artwork and wind chimes in theirs; others simply stretch plastic across some poles and staple it to the outside of their house and call it good. Either way, a greenhouse can be a sanctuary and a lovely place to begin the lives of new seeds.

COLD FRAMES are a consideration if you don't have access to a greenhouse. These are much smaller, often the width of a window. Taller in the back and shorter in the front, a cold frame is a box with a window for a lid. Often the lid can be held up with a simple stick. Situate the cold frame on the south-facing side of your property and place seed trays in them, propping the lid open depending on the weather so the seeds stay relatively warm. Be sure to bring the seeds inside if it promises to be a cold night, and be careful of breakable glass. Lid alternatives include plastic stretched across a frame or clear polystyrene.

Don't feel that you can't be a gardener or start seeds without a greenhouse or a cold frame. You can also start seeds in trays spread out on newspaper in front of a large glass window. The plastic tray lids available at garden stores can be very effective; just make sure you place the tray on a flat surface, keep them watered regularly, and turn the tray every couple of days to keep the new seedlings growing tall. The seeds will be ready to transplant within weeks.

Trellises

A trellis can be a simple and functional way to grow and enjoy your herbs. Many people think of trellises for vegetables and flowers, but they come in handy for herbs as well, especially hops and roses and for tall plants that sometimes need support, such as mallow, hibiscus, and valerian. Simply build a vertical box with two-by-four lengths of wood and zigzag string up and down so the herbs have something to cling to. If your trellis is sturdy, you can use it year after year for pole beans, cucumbers, and gourds. Hops, which are a medicinal herb useful as a sedative to promote sleep and as a bitter herb for digestion, will grow and produce prolifically one year and then the vines die back and the hops sprout the next year from new vines, meaning the trellis must be cleared off annually. This is easy if you've used string.

A trellis can be an imaginative focal point in your garden and can be a nice way to bring herbs into the vegetable garden or vegetables into the herb garden. Either way, this is an investment in both the productivity of your garden and its appeal, as it helps add a vertical element to an otherwise horizontal playing field.

Be Purposeful

When creating your growing space, whether it's a garden or a small porch with a pot or even a sunny windowsill, be purposeful in your intent. Slow down and enjoy the process so that gardening becomes less of a chore or a to-do list and more of a peaceful getaway, an activity you prize and a place you like to be. Let your growing space be a sanctuary where you can sit down with the plants, tiptoe over to your favorite flowers, and enjoy the sun on your face. If possible, be barefoot in your garden. A sense of mindfulness will help you grow your garden—and your enjoyment of herbs—as much as any fence or trellis.

• EXERCISE 1 •

Creating a Growing Space

STEP 1: **Envision the Purpose of Your Growing Space.** Will it be a kitchen herb garden? A garden for making herbal medicines? Will it attract butterflies? Do you primarily want it for cut flowers? Will you also grow vegetables, and do you want to supplement your meals with food and herbs from this garden? Decide what makes the most sense to you. It's possible to grow medicinal herbs alongside vegetables, but since many herbs are biennial or perennial and most vegetables are annual, it makes sense to grow them in separate areas of the garden. For this reason, I have a large medicinal herb garden with no fence around it, then inside a fenced area I grow vegetables.

STEP 2: **Next, Consider Garden Design.** There are so many ideas to choose from: you can create gardens planted in the shape of a giant keyhole, cross, crescent moon, etc. I know one woman who planted an Artemis garden, with only herbs in the Artemesia family; these are silvery plants that have a certain magic about them and the garden casts a silver-blue hue. Another woman planted a spiral garden with themes of life stages, incorporating flowers and herbs that were symbolic. Another friend planted a pizza garden filled with herbs and vegetables that she wanted to cook on her pizzas. Also, an array of potted plants of various sizes arranged on your porch or balcony can be beautiful and convenient.

STEP 3: **Prepare Your Space and Gather Your Seeds and Seedlings.** Prepare beds, digging as deep as you can, or prepare pots in an array of sizes. Seeds for fennel, nettle, catnip, calendula, holy basil, and valerian are easy to come by, and these plants grow well from seed. Other herbs, such as motherwort, thyme, oregano, anise hyssop, and lemon balm, are very easy to get as tiny seedlings from friends in the early spring. Because these herbs self-seed rampantly, they produce numerous babies that are easy to dig up with a small trowel; place them in the bed or pot of your choice. Other herbs, such as roses, rosemary, and lavender, are usually best purchased at a garden nursery. Buy the smallest ones you can find, as they grow quickly.

STEP 4: Now for the herbs! Which ones are you going to plant? There are literally hundreds of edible, medicinal, ornamental, and specialty herbs you could consider, but I suggest starting with just a handful that you feel drawn to or that you might be familiar with already. By beginning with five or six plants, you allow yourself time to get to know those plants well and discover how they grow in your area, how they like to be harvested, how they taste or smell, and how they act in the remedies you make. There are some great beginner herbs that will help you learn about plant medicine and plant gardening quickly and effortlessly, while other herbs require a little bit more of a learning curve. All are wonderful! Enjoy your explorations, and let your inner experimenter take over.

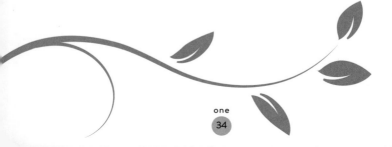

The Herb Lists

Here are some lists that will categorize a number of popular herbs and make it simple to decide which ones are best for you. The first presents easy and useful herbs to start with, which are some of the most common and popular herbs for beginners.

This is followed by unusual herbs to start with, which lists additional herbs to try if you're feeling adventurous and want to grow and use some helpful medicinals.

Next is herbs to allow to grow wild because wild harvesting is half the fun; these "weeds" show up in yards, meadows, and untamed places and are quite useful, so if you allow them to grow, you will be rewarded.

And finally, the list of herbs to avoid for your garden's sanity refers to wonderful plants that simply take over, quickly thwarting any hopes you had of a clean, organized, or even walkable garden. Some of these may be grown in a back corner or pot, but be vigilant about keeping them in check. This list also includes herbs you really never want to plant because they quickly become nuisances that cannot be eradicated and can actually destroy a garden.

Following the lists, you'll find an herbal properties chart that will help you even further in deciding which herbs you may want to plant and work with.

Easy and Useful Herbs to Start With

We will start with some basics that every beginner gardener should try. The basic criteria for including these here are straightforward; these herbs

- are easy to grow in most regions, and many can be grown in a pot on the windowsill;

- are safe for most people to use, and when there are contraindications (warnings), I will make note of them for you;

- can be made into simple remedies to be used for common health issues—for instance, most of these herbs can be brewed into simple teas, and they're used for common issues such as cough, runny noses, upset stomach, and wounds;

- make a great "starter" list, allowing you to get familiar with wonderful edible and medicinal plants in quick, easy, and creative ways.

If you grow five or six of these herbs, you will have a functional medicine cabinet in your garden or on your porch or balcony, and you will be able to address many illnesses, support most major body systems, and be of great service to your family and community.

The herbs in this list include anise hyssop, calendula, catnip, chamomile, elderberry, fennel, garlic, lavender, lemon balm, nettle, oregano, rose, rosemary, sage, spearmint, thyme, valerian, and yarrow.

Anise Hyssop
(Agastache foeniculum)

TYPE: perennial

HEIGHT: 4 to 6 feet

SMELL: sweet, fragrant, licorice

COLOR: blue-gray, light green; flowers are violet or pink

HABIT: Anise hyssop self-seeds rapidly and spreads like wildfire. It's easily transplanted when young and is easy to identify with its thick, fragrant blue-green leaves.

EDIBLE: Yes, the leaves can be tossed into salads or chewed fresh. Sprinkle the flower petals into salads and dressings.

MEDICINE: Anise hyssop is not the same plant as true hyssop, though they are both in the mint (Lamiaceae) family. Anise hyssop, also called giant hyssop or lavender hyssop, is very tall and woody and easy to grow in a garden; you'll find its babies emerging all over the garden in the spring, and they are easy to dig up and transplant where you want them.

As an aromatic herb, anise hyssop reliably performs in at least three ways in the body: it supports the respiratory system, the digestive system, and the nervous system. It is an expectorant, making it excellent for coughs. For this purpose, harvest the leaves and make a strong tea or prepare lozenges or cough drops using honey. (Also dry the leaves for use over the winter when coughs are probable.) For sluggish digestion, use anise hyssop infused into hot water for a tea, infused into honey for a syrup, or extracted into grain alcohol for a tincture to encourage stronger action by the gallbladder and ease diarrhea and intestinal cramps. For the nervous system, include anise hyssop in remedies for mild to moderate depression, irritability, and poor concentration. Anise hyssop is also vulnerary and can be included in topical wound remedies; its terpene (essential oil) content makes it useful for fighting infection.

TO HARVEST: individually harvest the leaves as needed

Calendula
(Calendula officinalis)

TYPE: annual

HEIGHT: 1 to 2 feet

SMELL: not noticeable

COLOR: green leaves with yellow or orange flowers

HABIT: Calendula grows on individual stalks, producing one or several flowers per stalk. Grow it in a row or sow it thickly in a small bed where you can easily reach the flowers.

EDIBLE: Yes, the petals: toss them in salads.

MEDICINE: Calendula, or pot marigold, has a long history of use, especially in European herbal traditions. It is prized as a skin remedy, and I've had extremely good results using it with people suffering with eczema, psoriasis, and other skin conditions. An oil infused with calendula flowers turns bright gold and can be used as-is or warmed with beeswax to create an ointment. Apply calendula oil to burns, wounds, sensitive and dry skin, chafed skin, allergic rashes, and to baby's bottom. Calendula is antimicrobial and will fight infection, and it makes an excellent addition to first aid ointments. Tinctured calendula can be used for influenza and other illnesses where additional immune support is needed.

TO HARVEST: Use your finger to pluck individual flower blossoms, but be aware your fingers will get very sticky. Remove individual petals from the flower head, place these in a jar, and cover with oil or ethyl alcohol.

Catnip

(Nepeta cataria)

TYPE: biennial

HEIGHT: 2 to 4 feet

SMELL: minty

COLOR: gray-green, silvery

HABIT: Catnip grows as a weedy, stalky mound; it tends to grow straight up but will be lazy and grow horizontally and diagonally if given the chance.

EDIBLE: Yes, but too dry and mealy to be palatable.

MEDICINE: Catnip is one of my favorite plants and one that seems to be largely ignored by many herbalists. Most people are familiar with catnip as "catmint," the herb that excites cats. (Other herbs are called catmint, too, though *Nepeta cataria* is the one loved by felines.) Many cats are stimulated by the smell of catnip and enjoy chasing the stalks when you use it as a toy or batting around toys stuffed with dried catnip leaves. Oddly, eating catnip leaves (instead of just smelling them) tends to sedate cats. Similarly, ingesting catnip leaves or a tea made from them will sedate people, and it's used in traditional herbal medicine as a very mild sedative. Its scent is minty and evocative, with a little sweetness and a little muskiness. It boasts very soft little leaves and is easy for children to harvest, and it is one of my most-used children's herbs. It's very safe, quite calming, makes a delicious tea, and is soothing to the nervous system.

Catnip, calendula, and chamomile are my go-to herbs for pregnant women and mothers with infants. These herbs are safe, versatile, and effective for a wide range of issues for both mother and baby. Catnip, being a mint, is a tasty herb, especially for those needing assistance sleeping, since it is calming and gently sedative. Together, catnip and chamomile make a wonderful bedtime tea for children, and it's one of those herbs that is easy to gather, so children feel invested in harvesting the leaves and making their own remedy with it.

Catnip is also a mild vulnerary, so it makes a useful rinse for a baby's cut or wound; sometimes an infant's fingernails grow in very sharp and they scrape themselves with their tiny fingers. A simple rinse of strained catnip tea (or calendula, sage, or elderflower) drizzled onto the skin will quickly heal the wound, especially if it is on the baby's face. Catnip is also an aromatic, meaning it will reliably support digestion, respiratory function, and the nervous system. Use it for upset tummies, nausea during pregnancy, gas, indigestion, cough, and congestion in both the upper and lower respiratory systems.

TO HARVEST: Pull up the entire plant and hang it to dry or snip off branches and then strip the leaves into a bag. Use both the leaves and the flowers, but harvest the leaves before they begin to shrink and dry up near the end of the season.

Chamomile
(Matricaria recutita)

TYPE: perennial

HEIGHT: 1 to 2 feet

SMELL: heady, aromatic, fragrant

COLOR: green or gray-green; tufts of white flowers atop dense stalks

HABIT: chamomile likes to grow in mounds or clusters; it makes a dense bed of dozens of plants and likes to grow close together

EDIBLE: not as a food, but it makes a lovely tea

MEDICINE: Chamomile is well-regarded as a safe, soothing, and delightful herb, often used as a calming or sedative remedy for those who can't sleep. It has been a favorite for centuries for its lovely flavor, full mouthfeel when brewed as a hot tea, easy growing habit, and fragrance. Chamomile is a favorite of children; I like to combine it with catnip for a soothing cup of tea at bedtime.

 Because chamomile is related to ragweed, use caution if you have hayfever or are allergic to ragweed.

TO HARVEST: snip the flowers and use them fresh in teas or dry them on a screen or in a dehydrator

Elderberry
(Sambucus nigra, S. Canadensis)

TYPE: perennial

HEIGHT: 8 to 20 feet

SMELL: not noticeable except when the leaves are
rubbed—they emit a rank smell

COLOR: The leaves are dark green and the flowers
are creamy white. Cultivated elderberries exist,
with a variety of colors. For instance, Japanese
elder has dark purple leaves and pink flowers.

HABIT: Elderberry is a large shrub or small tree,
and it likes to keep its feet wet and its head
in the sun. Elder likes wet, marshy areas near
creeks, swamps, or beaches, and they often
grow in groves. The trunk can get quite large,
and this sturdy tree can hold up many branches
supporting hundreds of flower and fruit heads.
Small trees can be easily accessed; larger trees
require ladders.

EDIBLE: Yes, elders are known for their tasty fruits
and lovely edible flowers. The fruits are tasty
when they're cooked; raw elderberries are not

very pleasant. They cook well with blueberries and make excellent pies and cobblers. The flowers can be infused into honeys. The whole flower head can be dipped into batter and fried. They make a lovely addition to teas, ice cubes, salads, and desserts, where their creamy color and fairy-like quality can be admired.

MEDICINE: Elders are ancient trees that have long held a solid place in the traditional medicinal repertoire of many cultures. Many lovely and haunting myths and stories surround the elder tree; she is called Hulda Mutter (Elder Mother) in Scandinavian myth, and people are warned they must ask permission from the tree before they harvest any part. Other stories caution that you can know a witch because she grows an elder tree outside her door, while others advise that you can keep witches away by growing an elder tree outside your door. The trees are native to both Europe and North America and have been used for multiple purposes for hundreds of years.

Let's start with the elder's flowers. In the spring the white flowers will form in heads—

umbels—that hang down and are easy to snap off with your fingers. Collect these heads and fill your tincture jars with the fresh flowers. The flowers are anti-inflammatory and soothing to hot, inflamed skin (such as a burn or poison ivy), and they are traditionally used for upper respiratory infections, sinus congestion, and fever. They are incredibly mild and very safe, making them ideal as a cold and flu remedy for children. I like to combine elderflowers with thyme, catnip, calendula, and sage for colds and flu, especially where there are sniffles, congestion, or earache or ear infection.

Elderberries form after the flowers, like any fruit. The berry of the elder tree is also used for the respiratory system—specifically for the lungs, the lower respiratory system. It has long been prized as a cough syrup because it is expectorant and anti-inflammatory and very soothing to lungs that have been upset with hacking coughs. Elderberries also support the immune system in fighting infection.

Elderberries are easy to harvest (snip off the whole head and then use your fingers to strip the berries from the roughage, if desired). For tinctures, leaving bits of the stem and stalk on the berries is fine, but for cobblers, remove as much as you can. Squash or mash them with the back of a spoon, or squeeze them between your hands to release some of the juice, then tincture or make into a syrup (see chapter 3 for instructions). I often combine elderberries with thyme, garlic, pleurisy root, mullein, elecampane, anise hyssop, or sage when making a cough remedy.

Finally, use the leaf of the elder tree for topical ointments. Harvest the fresh leaf at any time during the season; chop it coarsely, place it in a glass canning jar, and cover with olive oil. Leave this to steep on a dark, cool pantry shelf for two to four weeks, then strain and use as-is or add one-fourth cup chopped beeswax to every cup of oil, heat slowly, and pour into salve jars. This makes an excellent remedy for burns, cuts, bruises, and all manner of skin abrasions. Combine the elder leaf in the jar with herbs such as yarrow leaf, sage, mint, anise hyssop, plantain, wild geranium, or St. John's wort leaf and flower when making a first aid ointment.

TO HARVEST: Using your fingers, snip off the entire
flower head or the entire berry head and drop
them into a bag. Dry the flowers or berries for
later use, freeze the berries, or use everything
fresh. For the leaves, snip them off with your
fingers and use immediately.

Fennel
(Foeniculum vulgare)

TYPE: perennial, depending on zone

HEIGHT: 4 to 6 feet

SMELL: pleasant, sweet, licorice

COLOR: leaves can be green or bronze, flowers are
generally yellow

HABIT: In warm climates fennel spreads readily
and grows wild. In cooler climates it can act as
an annual and often is much shorter than wild
fennel. Harvest the seeds at the end of the season
and spread them to increase your yield.

EDIBLE: Yes, fennel is considered a vegetable and
spice plant, with the bulb, leaves, and seeds

included in cuisines around the world. The flowers are also used for flavoring.

MEDICINE: Fennel is carminative, making it an excellent herb for digestive illnesses such as indigestion, cramps, gas, and bloating. It is anti-inflammatory, easing pelvic congestion and other internal and external inflammation. Many cultures use fennel seeds as an after-dinner treat to aid the body in digestion. Use fennel leaves and seeds in respiratory remedies as a mild expectorant, combining it with thyme or elderberry. Fennel is also a galactagogue, increasing both the quality and quantity of breastmilk for nursing mothers.

TO HARVEST: Collect the leaves and chop them, or snip off the entire flower head once it's gone to seed and place it in a bag. Crush the seeds before adding them to your tincture.

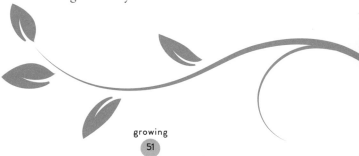

Garlic
(Allium sativa)

TYPE: annual, sometimes a recurring annual

HEIGHT: 2 to 4 feet

SMELL: not noticeable; slightly garlicky when rubbed

COLOR: green leaves, white or speckled flower head

HABIT: Bulbs produce a straight stalk with long slender leaves, then scapes. The scape is the stalk that will support the flower, but before it flowers the scape is tender and succulent, and it makes an excellent food, either sautéed or processed into pesto. Once the scape hardens, it is too late to use it, and the plant will flower. Cutting the scape is desired if you want the plant to focus its energy on the bulb. The bulb is composed of individual cloves, each of which is wrapped in its own papery skin, which must be peeled off before using. A clove can be planted to grow a new garlic plant.

EDIBLE: Yes, the bulb (raw or cooked) and the scape (processed into pesto or sautéed). Also the flower petals can be sprinkled into salads, etc.

MEDICINE: Garlic has been a multipurpose plant for centuries. It is used medicinally to treat a range of illnesses and infections, it is used as a food in cuisines around the world, and it is considered a type of spice or condiment, being ground into a powder and sprinkled onto foods as a flavoring. It can be a tricky plant to grow, as the bulbs can rot or not grow very large, and if you don't cut the flowering scapes in time, then you'll get no bulb at all because the plant will put its energy into flowers instead of the bulb. Regardless, garlic is worth it. The medicine is primarily antimicrobial: garlic fights fungal, bacterial, viral, and parasitic infections. Use both the garlic bulb and the flowering scapes in your remedies using vinegar or water, but avoid making infused oils for topical or internal use as these, in my experience, turn rancid very quickly and can burn the skin or make you sick. It's best to use garlic medicine fresh as a food; in certain remedies, such as a remedy to fight influenza, many herbalists will call for garlic to be consumed with juice. This means you should mince the fresh garlic finely and place a tiny amount, such as a quarter teaspoon, in a small glass of juice, perhaps along with other remedies such as apple cider vinegar or a dab of cayenne pepper, and drink it down in a couple of gulps. This keeps the garlic from burning the throat or upsetting the stomach. You may also make an infused vinegar or an oxymel with garlic (see chapter 3). Otherwise, plan your meals with garlic included as a food ingredient; this is the best way to ingest garlic for medicinal purposes.

TO HARVEST: Use scissors to snip off the scape; feel the stalk and determine where it is tender and where it starts to get firm—you want only the tender part. For the root, dig up in the fall after all aerial parts have died back and cure in a cool, dark place.

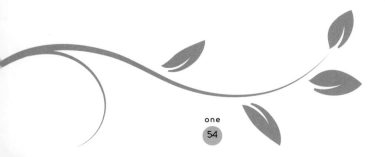

Lavender
(Lavandula spp.)

TYPE: perennial

HEIGHT: 12 to 18 inches

SMELL: lovely, fragrant, heady

COLOR: gray-green foliage, sometimes with a blue cast, sometimes silvery; flowers are light to dark purple

HABIT: Grows in a low, full mound and sends up spikes that can be short or very tall. Can be divided (cleaved).

EDIBLE: Yes, but because it is rather woody, it is not very palatable eaten whole. Try it in tea, and try flavoring other foods with it, such as infusing it in sugar, honey, vinegar, and milk. It can also be sprinkled lightly into salads and baked into breads and muffins. Also, sprinkle the tiny flowers into ready-made granola and lightly over waffles and pancakes.

MEDICINE: Lavender has centuries of use behind it throughout many countries and cultures. Because of its lovely aroma, it is a favorite for romance as well as scented goods for the household. It contains saponins that suds up when washed; the word *lavender* is a cognate of *laundry*. It is soothing to the skin and can be used on burns. Medicinally, lavender is considered soothing to the nerves, and many people find inhaling the scent will calm them and ease anxiety. Some people find the scent too stimulating, and it may cause headaches for them. I like to add a little dried lavender to tea blends that contain nettle, lemon balm, spearmint, ginger, or catnip; its flavor is a bright spot in a beverage, and the colorful flowers are beautiful in dried teas or potpourri. Lavender makes an excellent infused honey, transferring its flavor quickly and easily to honey overnight in a covered pot. Strain and use the honey in teas and on biscuits and toast.

TO HARVEST: Snip the base of the stalk near the bottom of the mound, then strip the leaves and flowers off with your fingers. The leaves are very resinous and woody and difficult to chop.

Lemon Balm
(Melissa officinalis)

TYPE: perennial

HEIGHT: 12 to 18 inches

SMELL: lemony, fresh, citrusy

COLOR: Leaves are medium green; flowers are tiny and light blue. In full sun the leaves tend to be very small and have a yellowish hue; grown in the shade, the leaves are broader and take on a deeper, richer green.

HABIT: This plant grows in a low, full mound and will self-seed and spread, popping up everywhere.

EDIBLE: Yes, the young, tender leaves can be tossed into a salad or brewed into a tea.

MEDICINE: Lemon balm is a lovely herb for the apothecary. Its leaves have many uses that make it a reliable support for anxiety and stress; it is calming without being sedative, though a very strong tea can be sedative, especially when combined with other sedative herbs such as valerian, hops, or catnip. Lemon balm is traditionally used to ease our mind's reaction to stress. Many people find it helps them focus, and those with ADD/ADHD attest to its value in helping them concentrate or ignore background stimuli so they can be present in the moment. Take lemon balm as a delicious tea (infusion), as an infused honey, and as capsules, tincture, vinegar, syrup, ice cubes, and poured into the bath (all of these remedies, except capsules, will be described in chapters 3 and 4). Lemon balm is also vulnerary, meaning it supports wound healing and is often included in wound salves and first aid ointments. Lemon balm is antiviral, so it makes a good addition to lip balms as a remedy for herpes simplex. Note that lemon balm can be contraindicated for those with hypothyroidism. Use with caution or avoid completely if you have hypothyroid disease or low blood pressure.

TO HARVEST: Snip off a branch and, using the fingers, strip the leaves off from the tip to the base. Discard the branch and chop the leaves for use.

Nettle
(Urtica dioica)

TYPE: perennial

HEIGHT: 4 to 8 feet

SMELL: not noticeable

COLOR: dark green

HABIT: Spreads by seeds and roots; will run rampant. Stings on contact, so plant it where it won't be brushed against easily. Use caution around children.

EDIBLE: Yes, nettle is a great food source. The leaves can be cooked like turnip greens—sauté them in a pan with oil, salt, and pepper. Steam or boil the leaves to add to soups, stews, and lasagna, or place a handful of fresh leaves into a food processor and create a dip with cream cheese and chives. Layer fresh leaves on top of pizza before it goes into the oven so that when it comes out it is cooked and slightly crisp. Try mixing nettle leaves with parsley and basil to make a pesto using olive oil and garlic; it's best to dry the nettle first or steam it. The seeds can be collected and baked on a cookie sheet, then sprinkled onto salads, granola, oatmeal, and vegetables.

MEDICINE: The word *nettle* comes from *needle*; this plant is covered in tiny, sharp, hollow needles that attach to a sac filled with histamine and formic acid—the same acid used by fire ants to deliver their sting. When you brush against the plant, the sac squeezes and pushes the histamine and formic acid through the hollow needle to inject it into your skin. This is the plant's protective mechanism; to use the plant, we must deactivate the sting. We can do this in two ways: cook the leaves or dry them. We cannot eat the fresh leaves without doing one of these two things. Fortunately, once we cook or dry the leaves, nettle is an incredibly nutritious food source, high in many minerals (including iron, calcium, and phosphorous) and vitamins (especially vitamin A). It is especially useful for micronutrient deficiency, giving a boost to those of us who are undernourished due to illness, pregnancy, stress, or poor soil and agriculture conditions.

Medicinally, nettle is a mineral and vitamin powerhouse, and it is also directly useful for certain conditions. Its iron content, for instance, makes it useful for anemia, which is often experienced by women with heavy menstrual cycles or endometriosis. However, nettle is high in vitamin K, making it necessary to avoid nettle for a week or so before having surgery, and resuming a week or so afterwards.

Nettle is mildly laxative, making it ideal for pregnant women experiencing constipation or for anyone with stuck bowels. If, on the other hand, you are having diarrhea, you will want to avoid nettle. It is also diuretic, so be sure to tell people who are using nettle tea or other remedies made with nettle that they may feel a more urgent need to go to the bathroom. Nettle seed and root are the subject of many tests for their apparent use in supporting men with benign prostatic hypertrophy and enlarged prostate.

Nettle makes a delicious, smooth tea that is silky on the mouth and has a full green flavor. It combines well with spearmint for digestion, lemon balm for calming nerves, and alfalfa, violet, and oat straw or oats milky tops for building strong bones, hair, and teeth.

TO HARVEST: see exercise 2 on page 137

Oregano
(Oreganum vulgare)

TYPE: perennial

HEIGHT: 12 to18 inches

SMELL: woodsy, resinous, minty

COLOR: dark green leaves with spikes of tiny purple blossoms

HABIT: Oregano grows in a mound and spreads as a mat, meaning it is a dense population of plants rather than individuals. A mat of oregano can grow several feet in every direction, and it is easy to dig out a section of this mat and replant it elsewhere. Oregano sends up soft spikes of flowers that look cloud-like above the green mat. Because of its growing habit, it is a good plant to place next to a rock wall, a rock stairway, or a fence.

EDIBLE: Yes, oregano is often dried and used as a culinary spice. The fresh leaves and blossoms are edible, but drying this herb brings out its flavor.

MEDICINE: Very similar to thyme (see below), oregano is used to counter infection, fight bacteria, and as an expectorant in cough remedies. I like to use oregano in first aid ointments as it is an excellent wound healer. It keeps infection at bay and can be used in ointments, poultices, and compresses.

TO HARVEST: Using your hands, gather as many stalks as possible and snip them from the base with scissors. Collect the stalks in a bag or basket, then hold each stalk upside down to strip its leaves off. Use the leaves and blossoms to make remedies; discard the stems.

Rose
(Rosa rugosa, R. spp.)

TYPE: perennial

HEIGHT: 4 to 6 feet

SMELL: sweet, fragrant

COLOR: Leaves are generally dark green; flowers can be white, cream, pink, red, etc. After the rose flowers, the petals die back to expose the growing fruit, called the hip. This grows into a small round fruit that is dark or bright red.

HABIT: Roses tend to grow into large mounds or shrubs; I've seen wild rose bushes the size of trees. The rose vines will use other trees and branches as supports. Roses in the garden must be pruned and usually have thorns. Cut the canes, or stems, back close to the ground every fall.

EDIBLE: Yes, the flower petals and the hips—the rose's fruits—are edible. Much like an apple grows on an apple tree after the blossom has died back, the hip grows on a rose bush after the rose petals fall away. The hips are high in vitamin C and usually have a strongly sour or tart flavor; many people value rose hip jelly for its tartness. Rose hips require steeping for 10 to 12 minutes; the tea will become very tart as the ascorbic acid is released. Rose petal jam is also a favorite of jelly connoisseurs because of its mildness and is considered a delicacy, and rose petals make a lovely tea.

MEDICINE: I consider roses a medicine for the heart, often giving them to friends and clients experiencing grief, sadness, or loss. Roses are a complementary medicine for anxiety and also for cardiovascular issues resulting in a weak heart or inefficient vessels and arteries, though they are a very mild medicine. Generally, their use is in the emotional realm as they assist a person in strengthening their "heart" through self-determination, self-confidence, and forgiveness. Roses tend to be cooling, helping those who are angry or hot-headed to calm down and regroup. Roses are wonderful for children experiencing pain, loss, grief, and trauma. Roses should be considered as aromatherapy for elders in nursing homes and for those in treatment facilities for addiction. Rose petals can be made into a tea (infusion), ice cubes, honeys, syrups, and eaten in oatmeal, topped on toast, baked into breads and muffins, cooked in puddings with rice or tapioca, and also used topically as a lotion,

cream, paste, or face mask. Fresh petals can be
sprinkled into the bathtub, and dried petals can
be rolled into incense. Rose hips can be cooked
and made into jams and preserves or tinctured.

TO HARVEST: Using gloves, individually harvest rose
petals or hips.

Rosemary
(*Rosmarinus officinalis*)

TYPE: perennial

HEIGHT: 2 to 8 feet

SMELL: minty, heady

COLOR: light green, gray-green

HABIT: large mound or shrub in warm climates;
small shrub in cooler climates

EDIBLE: Yes, though it is unpalatable as more than an
occasional spice. Rosemary stems are often used
as skewers when grilling meats and vegetables.

MEDICINE: Rosemary has been used for centuries
in a variety of ways: it is valued as the "herb of
remembrance," rightly so because its aroma is
not only uplifting but can directly affect memory

and clarity of thought. Its scent in aromatherapy is prized for this reason, and an occasional cup of rosemary tea, especially when blended with holy basil, can be refreshing and energizing. Rosemary is also antifungal and makes a valuable addition to first aid ointments. Rosemary spritzers (sprays) can be used not only on the skin but also as a home cleaning product. Avoid rosemary during pregnancy and breastfeeding.

TO HARVEST: Snip the whole stalk and strip the leaves.

Sage
(Salvia officinalis)

TYPE: perennial

HEIGHT: garden sage is generally 2 to 4 feet, including flower spikes

SMELL: minty, acrid, strong

COLOR: gray-green, silvery green with purple flowers

HABIT: Sage grows in medium-sized mounds with full, thick leaves. When it flowers it opens up a bit, appearing more leggy and less full. Its flower spikes reach straight upward with purple or pink petals. It will die back in the winter and return in the spring.

EDIBLE: Yes, in tiny cooked amounts or infused into butter.

MEDICINE: A key astringent, sage is parchy and dry. Use it for weepy sores and wet conditions such as poison ivy blisters, eczema, or pus-filled wounds. Use it internally for conditions such as diarrhea; a little will go a long way. Sage combines with tulsi as a general women's tonic, with turmeric for a brain tonic, and with yarrow for urinary tract infections, both topically and as a douche.

TO HARVEST: Snip the leaves off and pluck the flowers by using your fingers. Mince the leaves for a poultice or to infuse into oil, grain alcohol, or vinegar.

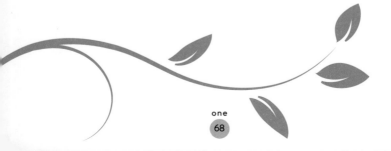

Spearmint
(Mentha spicata)

TYPE: perennial

HEIGHT: 1 to 2 feet

SMELL: minty, sweet

COLOR: light green, gray-green

HABIT: small mounds, or little "bursts" of growth; spreads from the roots

EDIBLE: Yes: chew on its own or add leaves to salad or grain dishes.

MEDICINE: Spearmint is highly aromatic, indicating its use in the respiratory system, the digestive system, and the nervous system. For the lungs, it is an expectorant, helping to expel mucus. Use it as a tincture or tea in the upper respiratory system for sinus congestion and infection, when the nose is clogged or runny, and when ear infection is present. It can be applied as a salve on the chest or under the nose for these purposes as well, since the aroma of the plant is healing. For digestion, spearmint is carminative, meaning it will ease an upset stomach, indigestion, flatulence, constipation, etc. Because of its high essential oil content, spearmint makes a delicious tea (quick brew) but is not appropriate for infusions (long brew). Use it to ease frazzled nerves, to provide energy and focus (without caffeine), and to give children a nice wake-up drink in the morning. Combine spearmint with nettle, ginger, and chamomile. Spearmint is cooler and sweeter than peppermint, which tends to be hotter and spicier; also, spearmint tends to focus on the core of the body (stomach and lungs), while peppermint tends to work on the extremities (hands, feet, and head).

TO HARVEST: Snip the whole stalk and strip the leaves.

Thyme
(Thymus vulgaris)

TYPE: perennial

HEIGHT: low to the ground, often a creeper

SMELL: woodsy, minty, fresh

COLOR: light to dark green foliage, with light to dark purple flowers

HABIT: Thyme forms low mounds with tiny leaves, producing tiny light purple blossoms on woody branches. Both thyme and oregano put out spikes of flowers, though thyme is not as easy to cleave, or split, as oregano.

EDIBLE: Yes, but it's too woody to be palatable.

MEDICINE: Thyme is strongly antimicrobial and is renowned for killing bacterial and fungal infections on contact. The leaves and flowers are strong wound healers and should be included in first aid ointments, wound liniments, and rinses for infections. Include thyme in respiratory formulas because it has a strong affinity for the lungs and the sinuses; thyme is an excellent remedy for cough and bronchial congestion. Thyme makes an effective and delicious infused honey and infuses well into apple cider vinegar. I like to include thyme in my fire cider vinegars along with garlic, horseradish, onion, cayenne, turmeric, and other spices and spicy herbs. If you have access to distillation equipment, thyme makes a wonderful hydrosol and essential oil.

TO HARVEST: Harvest just before flowering or
    during flowering. Cut the stalk at the base and
    strip the leaves and flowers from it to use in your
    remedies.

Valerian
(Valeriana officinalis)

TYPE: biennial

HEIGHT: 4 to 6 feet

SMELL: fragrant, sweet (the flowers, that is; the root
    smells of dirty feet)

COLOR: green foliage with creamy white flower
    heads

HABIT: Valerian grows tall from a single stalk with
    multiple branches, holding up numerous flower
    heads. It forms a mass of strikingly toothed
    leaves at its base the first year, and the second
    year it sends up stalks that often grow head-high
    or taller.

EDIBLE: no

MEDICINE: Valerian, in addition to being beautiful and fragrant, has two primary uses that make it functionally useful for the medicine cabinet. First, it is a sedative; the root has long been used to support healthy sleep, and it tinctures well. Because of the root's unfortunate smell, it doesn't make the best tea. However, the flowers are also mildly sedative, and they smell lovely; add them to teas with chamomile, hops, catnip, or lemon balm. Secondly, the root and the flowers are strongly anti-inflammatory. The flowers are actually quite strong in this regard and make an excellent analgesic oil for arthritis, sore muscles, and tight joints. I've had very good luck combining valerian flowers with clove and lavender for rheumatic complaints, as well as infusing them into an oil and turning them into a salve to be rubbed on painful shoulders and joints.

TO HARVEST: The flowers are easy to harvest: snip them with your fingers or with snippers and infuse them directly into an oil. The root can be dug up in the fall after the flowers have died back; spray the roots off with a hose (they will be spaghetti-like, thin, and numerous). Chop them and let them dry thoroughly before steeping them in a carrier oil such as olive.

Yarrow
(Achillea millefolium)

TYPE: perennial

HEIGHT: 12 to 18 inches

SMELL: slightly acrid, pleasant, strong

COLOR: Wild yarrow generally has bright green leaves and white flowers. Cultivars can be of many colors; my cultivated yarrow has silvery gray leaves and yellow flowers. Other flower colors include pink, violet, and red.

HABIT: Upright stalks stiffly hold up dry flower heads. The leaves are soft and relaxed and will form a low, full mound the first year, with the stalks rising up the second year. Individual yarrows can be easily transplanted; mounds can be cleaved and halved. It's not necessarily a spreader as it tends to stay where you put it.

Wild yarrow is a small, spindly herb that works to poke its way up between other more robust plants in a field or roadside. Cultivated yarrow, on the other hand, tends to grow lush and full and can be divided every year or so and moved elsewhere.

EDIBLE: Yes, the leaves are edible but bitter, so only a small amount can be consumed at a time. The flavor is generally too strong to consider it a food.

MEDICINE: Yarrow is a potent medicinal plant with many actions and is a medicine cabinet in itself. Yarrow is diuretic (will increase the volume of urine), diaphoretic (will induce perspiration), antimicrobial (a catch-all term meaning it is antibacterial, antifungal, antiparasitic, and antiviral), bitter, and more. Use yarrow for urinary tract infections, to relieve pain, and to reduce inflammation.

Because it is bitter, it is a digestive stimulant, easing bloating, constipation, and gas. It is a diaphoretic, especially when drunk as a hot tea—helpful for colds or when fever needs to be reduced.

Yarrow is an exceptional antibacterial herb, killing germs both internally and externally, and because it is a strong diuretic (increasing the urge to pee and the quantity of urine), it makes an excellent treatment for urinary tract infections.

Use yarrow in topical wound remedies and first aid ointments and oils. The leaf is styptic (a very strong remedy to stop bleeding), helping staunch blood flow on the surface of the skin. It is readily astringent and helpful for wounds of all sorts, weeping sores, poison ivy, and as a soak for the perineum after childbirth and as a rinse for the baby's cut cord. (See exercise 28, making a spit poultice, and exercise 30, making a regular poultice). Include yarrow in first aid remedies, flu tinctures, and sitz baths for postpartum care.

TO HARVEST: Snip the leaves from the base of the plant or snap off the entire stalk, hold it upside down, and strip the leaves off, collecting them as well as the flowers. I find the leaves are more effective for external remedies, but I include the flowers as well as the leaves in tinctures.

The Three Easiest Herbs

If you're just beginning to garden and feeling over-
whelmed, the list of easy and useful herbs to start
with should be helpful. But if you want to narrow
down your choices even more, the top three on that
list are lemon balm, spearmint, and yarrow. If you're
worried about safety, these are among the safest.
They are also versatile—each of these can be used
internally and externally for a wide range of remedies. These three perennials are also very easy to
grow: in pots or in a garden, they are likely to thrive.

Unusual Herbs to Start With

Once you've grown confident growing and using herbs such as catnip, lemon balm, and spearmint, these less well-known herbs will add some new interest. Many of them, such as mallow, black cohosh, and borage, sport beautiful flowers and will add intrigue and color to your garden or plant pots.

These unusual herbs also up your game in creating remedies for a variety of illnesses or conditions; rather than being gentle tonics, as most of the easy herbs are, many of these are a bit stronger and can address a wide range of illnesses. For instance, motherwort is a bitter herb that is wonderful for digestion; it also supports healthy cardiovascular action and eases anxiety and fear. Black cohosh can be enjoyed simply for its striking upright flower stalk, but it is also a traditional remedy for women going through menopause; its root is tinctured. It is known in China as dong quai.

Enjoy exploring these plants, many of which may become your favorites in the years to come. This list includes angelica, black cohosh, black cumin, borage, cannabis, elecampane, ginger, hibiscus, holy basil, hops, mallow, motherwort, self-heal, and turmeric.

Angelica

(Angelica archangelica, A. sinensis)

TYPE: biennial

HEIGHT: 4 to 8 feet

SMELL: lightly fragrant

COLOR: dark green or purple stalk and foliage, purple or pink flowers

HABIT: Angelica generally stands up straight and tall, growing as an upright stalk with large showy leaves and giant umbels.

EDIBLE: Yes, angelica has a long history of being eaten as a food. Many parts of the plant are edible: the stem and leaf stalks, in particular, can be sliced and rolled in sugar to make a candy. The leaves can be eaten raw and tossed into salads, and the flowers can be sprinkled into salads or baked into muffins. Angelica seeds can be nibbled fresh, sprinkled into salads, or candied.

MEDICINE: As an aromatic, angelica can be counted on for three distinct health purposes (as can all aromatics): respiratory, digestive, and nervous system medicines.

For respiratory ailments, use angelica for wet and dry coughs (especially as a tea), and for both upper and lower congestion. Include angelica in remedies for sinusitis and stuffy/runny nose as well as for bronchial congestion. Because the essential oils will be inhaled, include angelica in any paste or ointment you make that is rubbed on the chest or the lips. Angelica combines well for respiratory issues with elderflower and elderberry, violet leaf, and thyme.

For digestive ailments—including gas, constipation, diarrhea, heartburn, and pain—include angelica tea or tincture in the remedy process. Angelica combines well with chamomile, spearmint, lemon balm, valerian flower, catnip, motherwort, and ginger for digestive issues.

For nervous system issues, angelica is a soothing and enlivening remedy that eases mild to moderate depression and feelings of heaviness or being "stuck." Combine angelica with St. John's wort, lemon balm, rose petal, and fennel.

TO HARVEST: The strongest medicine of angelica is in the root; dig up the plant in its first year or in the second year once the flowers and seeds have died back. Clean, chop, and tincture immediately. Also, experiment with the stem or stalk by chopping it and rolling it in sugar; this is a traditional candy that makes a great cough lozenge or digestive remedy.

Black Cohosh
(Actaea racemosa, formerly Cimicifuga racemosa)

TYPE: perennial

HEIGHT: 4 to 8 feet

SMELL: not noticeable

COLOR: green foliage with creamy white flowers

HABIT: Black cohosh grows on tall stalks from a broad, fluffy base. It can easily grow taller than most people, and its wispy flower heads will blossom and then droop, giving it a casual appearance on an otherwise formal plant. It can be planted either as the centerpiece of a garden or along other tall plants such as fennel, hollyhock, valerian, and tall species of bee balm. Black cohosh likes rich, moist soil and its native habitat is woodland, so it prefers shade, but it does well in full sun as long as the soil is good and it is watered frequently.

EDIBLE: no

MEDICINE: The root of black cohosh contains the medicinally active chemicals that are generally used for women's reproductive issues, especially childbirth. Black cohosh root is astringent (drying) and anti-inflammatory, and it is an expectorant, making it a valuable medicine to support the uterus during childbirth. (This is why it should be avoided by pregnant women who aren't at the childbirth stage yet.) Black cohosh is also a traditional remedy for menopause and hot flashes; many women find a tincture of black cohosh root is effective in easing hot flashes and reducing the symptoms of menopause. For those who are not pregnant, it can also be used for wet cough.

TO HARVEST: Dig up plants that are at least three years old, clean and chop the root, and tincture it.

Black Cumin
(Nigella sativa)

TYPE: annual

HEIGHT: 6 to 8 inches

SMELL: not noticeable

COLOR: flowers are bright blue or white

HABIT: self-seeds and spreads easily, produces feathery leaves on diminutive stalks

EDIBLE: The mature seeds inside the pod are edible.

MEDICINE: Also called love-in-a-mist, black cumin possesses seeds that are high in omega-3 fatty acids. These seeds can be crushed or eaten whole, added to smoothies, oatmeal, and other foods, or added to cosmetic preparations such as oils (to be infused and then strained out).

TO HARVEST: When the pod is dry and you hear the seeds shake inside, the pod is ready to break open. The seeds are incredibly tiny.

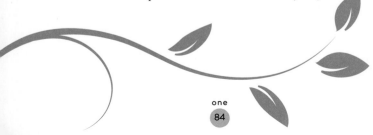

Borage
(Borago officinalis)

TYPE: annual

HEIGHT: 12 to 24 inches

SMELL: crushed leaves smell of cucumber

COLOR: flowers can be white, purple, pink, or blue

HABIT: grows as small individual plants, producing multiple flowers per plant

EDIBLE: Yes, the leaves, flowers, and seeds are all edible raw, having a sweet cucumber flavor. Many people like to put the starry, colorful flowers in ice cubes, and the leaves make a calming tea.

MEDICINE: Borage is traditionally the flower of courage, having been added to recipes for self-confidence for centuries. It is often included in cordials for this reason and also for its lightly sweet cucumber flavor. Topically, the leaves and flowers may be poulticed or used in ointments and oils because they are a reasonable vulnerary, though the leaves can be hairy and a compress may be more appropriate.

TO HARVEST: Using the fingers, snip off the leaves
and flowers as needed.

Cannabis
(Cannabis sativa, C. indica)

TYPE: annual

HEIGHT: 4 to 12 feet

SMELL: strong, fragrant, noticeable

COLOR: The entire plant is gray-green, sometimes
silvery. Different strains appear with leaves or
flowers that are blue, silver, orange, golden, or
purple.

HABIT: Cannabis tends to grow upwards in a straight
stalk, but it can be pruned to become bush-like.

EDIBLE: Yes, though generally it is not considered a
food.

Check with your local and state
authorities to determine the legal
status of cannabis where you live.

MEDICINE: If growing and using cannabis is legal
where you live, consider it as a healing remedy.

one
86

Cannabis is one of the most complex plants we know—chemically, botanically, culturally, and historically. Leaving aside its history and the politics surrounding it because it contains chemicals that are hallucinatory, we will focus simply on the medicinal aspects of the herb.

Traditionally, it is used as an antispasmodic and an anti-inflammatory, with well-known beneficial effects on spastic muscles and nervous tension. Cannabis supports those with epilepsy and other seizures, easing muscle control and making it a possible support for those with Parkinson's disease. Its anti-inflammatory effects support stiff muscles, wounds (topically), and perils of inflammation internally, including indigestion, endometriosis, fibroids and fibroid tissues, and arthritis.

As a nervine tonic, cannabis is complex, partly because while it is a prime nervous system relaxer, it is difficult to separate the nervous system benefits from a hallucinatory experience. Modern methods of hybridization, harvest, and processing are being developed to separate and distinguish these properties.

TO HARVEST: For antispasmodic relief, harvest the
buds and/or leaves and infuse them in a carrier
oil such as olive.

Elecampane
(Inula helenium)

TYPE: biennial

HEIGHT: 5 to 7 feet

SMELL: not noticeable

COLOR: green leaves, sometimes with a silvery or
blue hue, with yellow flowers

HABIT: Elecampane will grow as a fluffy mound
of long leaves its first year and will send up its
tall stalk the second year and produce flowers.
Sometimes it sends up several stalks and will
develop a habit of leaning and branching. The
flowers resemble small bright yellow sunflowers.

EDIBLE: no

MEDICINE: The most medicinal part of the plant is
the root, though the flowers can also be used;
if harvesting the root, wait until the end of the
growing season after the flowers have died away.

Elecampane is prized as a cough remedy—specifically as an antispasmodic, reducing spastic cough and easing the ability to breathe. I find this is most useful at night: taking a tincture of elecampane allows a child or adult to stop the dry, hacking coughs and sleep. When I use it, I feel my lungs relax and the constant impulse to cough is gone. It can be an odd sensation, especially since you can still feel the congestion in the lungs and you know the mucous is still there, but the cough has stopped. You sleep; in the morning take an expectorant such as pleurisy root to activate the lungs again and remove the phlegm. It's a strange remedy that has saved me and my children frequently, allowing everyone in the house to get much-needed sleep and recover from a cold or the flu.

Use elecampane in various ways: in a tincture with vodka, in a tincture with white wine, in a tincture with apple cider vinegar, and in a honey. After you've tinctured the chopped roots, you'll notice that the roots develop a white crystalline appearance; this is normal and to be expected. Let your tincture sit at least two months before using.

TO HARVEST: Dig up the plant in either its first year or in the second year well after the flowers have died back. Ideal times to harvest roots are at the end of the growing season and at a new moon.

Ginger
(Zingiber officinale)

TYPE: perennial in tropical areas such as Hawaii or southern Florida

HEIGHT: 2 to 4 feet

SMELL: not noticeable

COLOR: bright green leaves with yellow flowers; the root interior is bright yellow

HABIT: related to turmeric, ginger grows in warm, tropical climates as a small shrub or garden plant

EDIBLE: The root or rhizome is used as a spice in cuisines around the world. It is used fresh or dried as a condiment, cooked in candies, and minced or grated fresh into dishes. It is renowned for its fresh, zingy flavor and heat.

MEDICINE: As a food and medicine, ginger has been a favorite in many cultures for centuries. Its distinct flavor is prized in sauces, curries, main dishes, and beverages, and it is a staple in most markets and stores. Medicinally, ginger is a safe and well-known remedy, often used to ease stomachaches and nausea, even for children and during pregnancy in very small doses. Ginger is often included in cough remedies because it is a well-known circulatory stimulant and will get things moving, which is especially useful for stagnant conditions such as thick mucus congestion in the upper or lower respiratory systems. (It is for this reason that excessive ginger use can interfere with anticoagulant medications such as warfarin or aspirin.) For the same reason, people use ginger for arthritis, using it both internally as a tea or tincture and externally as a poultice, where it feels warming on the skin and penetrates to the muscles beneath.

TO HARVEST: Dig the root after the rest of the plant fades seasonally; ginger is "scalded" to keep it from resprouting, then cleaned and chopped. Commercial preparers boil the root, dry it,

then pound it. Gardeners can use the root
fresh, dry it, or tincture it/infuse it in grain
alcohol, vinegar, or other liquid. If infusing it in
oil, be aware that fresh ginger has a high water
content; allow the chopped root to wilt a bit on
newsprint before infusing it in oil.

Hibiscus
(Hibiscus sabdariffa, spp.)

TYPE: perennial

HEIGHT: 4 to 16 feet

SMELL: floral

COLOR: flowers are bright red; cultivars are white,
  pink, red, etc.

HABIT: upright flower stalk

EDIBLE: Yes, the sepals of *H. sabdariffa* are used in
  flavorings and beverages.

MEDICINE: *H. sabdariffa* makes a deliciously tart
  drink called roselle, often used to refresh and
  build stamina. The flowers and fruit are boiled
  to create a beverage with a similar tart and
  acidic flavor to the herb sorrel. Because it is

traditionally used to reduce blood pressure, some herbalists use the herb in combination with hypotensive medicines including garlic, hawthorn, and oatstraw.

TO HARVEST: Commercial preparers strip the calyx by hand, generally focusing on the stalk, which is prized as a fiber.

Holy Basil
(Ocimum tenuiflorum, O. sanctum)

TYPE: perennial in warm climates; annual in cooler climates such as New England

HEIGHT: 2 to 4 feet

SMELL: very fragrant, minty

COLOR: green or purple leaves; nondescript white or lilac flowers

HABIT: Holy basil has a thin stem that branches; overall, it is a light, sparse, woody little plant with small leaves. It self-seeds readily and is easy to grow from seed.

EDIBLE: Yes, the leaves may be sprinkled in salads.

MEDICINE: Holy basil is an entirely different plant than culinary basil, which is native to the Mediterranean. Holy basil is native to India and is known as tulasi or tulsi. It is a very sacred plant in Indian culture and religion, and it is used widely in ceremony. Holy basil is a featured herb in the Ayurvedic healing tradition, which is India's ancient science of medicine that combines diet, herbal remedies, yoga, and state of mind into its therapy. Holy basil is traditionally used for a wide variety of ailments, including bronchial, digestive, and nervous system issues. In western herbal medicine holy basil is renowned as a calming and relaxing herb, often included in teas to ease anxiety.

TO HARVEST: Snip the stem, turn it upside down, and in one motion strip the leaves and flowers from it. Collect these in a bag and use fresh or dried.

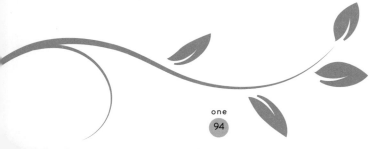

Hops
(Humulus lupulus)

TYPE: perennial

HEIGHT: Hops is a vine that climbs and needs
trellises or fences that allow it to reach 6 to 10
feet tall.

SMELL: not noticeable

COLOR: green vine with brown/red undertones;
greenish yellow strobiles

HABIT: Viney, drooping strobiles. Hops vines are
clingy, possessing hairs on the vines that cling to
fences and even to other plants. Hops will send
out vines that wrap themselves around other
nearby plants; you'll need to physically pull the
vines off and re-route them or trim them back.
New growth happens on new vines each spring,
so the old vines can be removed.

EDIBLE: no

MEDICINE: Hops have multiple medicinal actions,
including sedative (supporting sleep), bitter
(easing digestion), and galactagogue (increasing
breastmilk for nursing mothers). Hops have

a pleasant bitterness that can soothe stomach complaints; combine hops with other sedative herbs such as valerian or chamomile. Their bitterness makes them useful in brewing beer; when using hops for digestive issues, combine them with other bitter herbs such as motherwort, yarrow, or calendula, or with carminative herbs such as spearmint, catnip, and fennel. As a galactagogue (an herb that supports the production of breastmilk), hops are a gentle worker best combined with fennel, dill, spearmint, and bitter milk thistle, along with drinking lots of water and increasing the frequency of nursing.

TO HARVEST: When the strobiles have reached a light yellow color and a fluffy consistency, they are ready to snip off the vine. They are somewhat sticky and you will end up with a yellow sticky substance on your fingers. In the spring when new vines are sprouting from the ground, they may be dug up and transplanted.

Mallow

(Althea officinalis)

TYPE: perennial

HEIGHT: 2 to 4 feet

SMELL: lightly fragrant

COLOR: vibrant green, soft leaves; white or pink
flowers

HABIT: small upright stems that grow in narrow
clusters

EDIBLE: Yes, for centuries the flowers, leaves, and
roots have been eaten (fresh, fried, boiled, and
otherwise); the tender young leaves as well as
the flowers can be added to salads. The roots can
be chopped and boiled, as they are the original
source of our treats called "marshmallows."

MEDICINE: Mallow is both emollient and demulcent,
meaning it is soothing and cooling to tissues
both internally and externally. As an external
emollient, mallow leaves, flowers, and roots can
be processed (by chopping or poulticing) and
placed upon the skin, easing burns, cuts, and
inflammation. As an internal demulcent, a thick

tea of the leaves or roots can be ingested to ease and soothe symptoms associated with ulcers, heartburn, and indigestion, as well as spastic cough and burning throat issues. The root can be added to a syrup or lozenge to ease a sore throat.

TO HARVEST: The leaves are easy to harvest: snip them with your fingers and enjoy the soft, velvety feel of them on your skin. The roots can be dug up (harvesting the entire plant), cleaned, and chopped. Use fresh when possible.

Motherwort
(Leonurus cardiaca)

TYPE: biennial or perennial, depending on climate

HEIGHT: 2 to 6 feet

SMELL: not noticeable

COLOR: green leaves with pale purple flowers

HABIT: Motherwort will grow as a small single stalk or branch out, shrub-like. It is easily transplanted when small; it's easy to spot its deeply toothed leaves. Simply dig it up, keeping its little root ball intact as much as possible, and move it where you'd like it to be.

EDIBLE: Motherwort leaves are edible. I like to chew on a tiny leaf while I'm in the garden. They are bitter—to some, even unpalatable—but I like the bitterness and find it refreshing. The flowers can be sprinkled on salads, though I don't find much of a flavor to them.

MEDICINE: Motherwort is a medicine chest unto itself, offering many benefits from this simple yet complex plant. Use motherwort in three specific ways:

First, as a bitter for digestion, motherwort is an easy plant to include in digestive tinctures, syrups, and oxymels. Though it's too bitter to include in teas, motherwort makes a superb tincture with alcohol or vinegar, and its ease of use makes it useful for sudden indigestion, gas, bloating, and especially nervous indigestion issues that arise due to anxiety or fear. If you're supporting someone who gets an upset stomach before doing something scary (like taking a test), motherwort may be a good choice. It's also great for women whose digestion gets sluggish or volatile during the menstrual cycle. Because it's bitter, avoid this herb during pregnancy—though it's called motherwort (herb of the mother), it is primarily for mothers *after* the baby is born.

Second, motherwort is a nervine tonic to ease anxiety and feelings of panic. Its common name indicates it is for mamas who are stressed out caring for small children, who need extra energy, or who are feeling pangs of panic due to a wide range of reasons. A few drops of motherwort tincture on the tongue or a nibble of a fresh leaf will often relieve feelings of stress and the tightness in the chest that comes along with anxiety. Pair motherwort with St. John's wort, chamomile, catnip, or roses for nervous exhaustion.

Finally, motherwort is a heart tonic to support and strengthen cardiac function. Its Latin name means "heart of the lion," as it is traditionally used to support heart strength. Motherwort is a short-term remedy that can be used to support the heart during times of intense stress, fear, panic, or uncertainty. Use it for up to two weeks, along with hawthorn, rose, linden, garlic, and oats, to support heart health.

TO HARVEST: Using your fingers, snip the leaves off as needed. As the plant matures, it develops prickly spines along the stem that form in clusters, so gloves may come in handy. Young leaves are tender, while older leaves get woody; both are useful in medicine.

Self-Heal
(Prunella vulgaris)

TYPE: perennial

HEIGHT: 4 to 6 inches

SMELL: not noticeable

COLOR: dark green or purple leaves, light purple flowers

HABIT: Self-heal grows as a ground cover, forming a mat or appearing in small colonies that spread across a yard or garden.

EDIBLE: The tiniest leaves may be snipped and sprinkled in a salad, and the flower petals may be eaten as well.

MEDICINE: Also called heal-all, self-heal was traditionally considered a panacea, used for everything from cough to congestion to indigestion to headache. It serves as a support herb, boosting the strength of other herbs while not being quite strong enough to be the primary remedy. It can be included in first aid ointments for wounds (raspberries, scratches, scrapes, insect bites, and rashes) and in respiratory teas or tinctures for its mild action on both wet and dry coughs.

TO HARVEST: Snip the leaves and flowers with your fingers; if the plant gets mowed down, self-heal will grow back and you'll get another harvest.

Turmeric
(Curcuma longa)

TYPE: perennial in tropical areas such as Hawaii or southern Florida

HEIGHT: 1 to 2 feet

SMELL: not noticeable

COLOR: bright green leaves with brightly colored flowers; the root interior is bright orange

HABIT: Related to ginger, turmeric grows in warm, tropical climates as a small shrub or garden plant.

EDIBLE: The root is used as a spice. It can also be eaten fresh and has the taste and texture of a carrot.

MEDICINE: Warm and bitter, turmeric is an ancient herb originally called *terra merita*, "good earth," or more specifically "worthy land." Commonly used as a dye and a spice, turmeric is also a well-known remedy for aches, muscle tension, and arthritis. Recent research is revealing that turmeric is a brain tonic; the curcumin in the root support the body's natural process of protecting and nurturing brain cells, or neurons. It also strengthens the myelin sheath, the fatty layer surrounding the axon of the neuron that allows the potassium-sodium electrical charge to function. Without this, we develop diseases such as ALS (amyotrophic lateral sclerosis, multiple sclerosis, and Parkinson's). To this end, turmeric may prove to be a remedy for these diseases as well as for Alzheimer's and other dementias.

TO HARVEST: Dig the root after the rest of the plant fades seasonally; clean and chop. Commercial preparers boil the root, dry it, then pound it. Gardeners can use the root fresh, dry it, or tincture it/infuse it in oil.

Herbs to Allow to Grow Wild

Whether you actively garden or not, you will likely come across a number of wild plants that naturalize themselves in your yard or growing area. These are often beneficial and medicinal; rather than pull them up, allow them to flourish and harvest them seasonally. You will be rewarded with beauty, food, and medicine—all abundant and free.

Be sure to harvest from areas that are free from chemical contamination: avoid roadsides and beware of farms that spray chemicals on their crops. Also avoid areas beneath electric, power, and telephone lines, by telephone poles, and near golf courses that spray chemicals. Encourage your neighbors and nearby property owners to avoid chemicals and instead support natural mulch and organic options such as using horse manure fertilizer or managing insect pests with methods including crop rotation, companion planting, and herb-based sprays.

There are hundreds of beautiful and useful wild plants; to help the beginner discover the value of what is most likely to grow nearby, this list includes dandelion, jewelweed, plantain, pleurisy root, red clover, St. John's wort, violet, and yellow dock/burdock.

Dandelion
(Taraxacum officinale)

TYPE: perennial

HEIGHT: 6 to 12 inches

SMELL: not noticeable

COLOR: dark green leaves with reddish opaque stalks and bright yellow flowers

HABIT: Dandelion is a ground-loving plant; it begins with a basal rosette and sends up a hollow stalk with a bright yellow flower. Dandelions are hairless, which helps identify them, as chicory and other lookalikes have hairs on the stalks or leaves. Dandelion sends down a taproot and often grows in poor soil. Dandelions are beloved by bees; this is a great plant to allow to grow wild as it supports the local bee population.

EDIBLE: Yes, all parts of the plant are edible and nutritious. The blossom can be eaten raw or made into wine; the leaves are high in potassium and other minerals and can be eaten raw or cooked; the root is high in iron and can be chopped and sautéed.

MEDICINE: Dandelion has a wealth of medicine for such a diminutive "weed." The leaf is diuretic, giving it the nickname *pis-en-lit*, or "wet-the-bed"; dandelion can be included in cardiovascular formulas where a diuretic is needed. It is also bitter, stimulating digestion and useful in bitter formulas, and the root's iron content makes it valuable for anemia, menstruation, and as a general tonic. I like to infuse the whole herb (leaf, root, and blossom if it is in flower) in apple cider vinegar; this can be taken straight, used in salad dressings, or turned into an oxymel with honey (see exercise 20).

TO HARVEST: Snip individual leaves or use a trowel to dig the root.

Jewelweed
(Impatiens spp.)

TYPE: annual

HEIGHT: 2 to 6 feet

SMELL: not noticeable

COLOR: flowers are orange or yellow; leaves are
silvery green or bright green

HABIT: Jewelweed grows in moist, rich soil, often in
creeks and on creek banks where it can stay wet
and cool. The plant grows in a single stalk with
long, grasping reddish roots that perch above the
soil so that the bottom of the plant looks claw-
like.

EDIBLE: Yes, especially the new sprout in the spring.
The first two leaves can be snipped to eat raw
and are very sweet and tasty. The blossoms are
edible as well but are a bit parchy.

MEDICINE: Jewelweed is a very cooling, soothing
emollient for the skin and is the traditional
remedy for rashes and itches such as poison
ivy. Also called touch-me-not (when touched,
the ripe flowers will spring out their seeds),

jewelweed's primary medicine is found in its stalk. The stalk is hollow, and if the plant is large enough, it can be a couple of inches or more in circumference. Break open the stalk to find its juicy liquid; this relieves rashes and itch. Place the stalk and its liquid directly on the skin for immediate relief or chop the stalk into pieces and place them in a blender, then strain the liquid out. Store this liquid in an ice cube tray so that if poison ivy arises, you have little jewelweed ice cubes at the ready. I also like to chop the stalk into pieces and infuse them in a jar of witch hazel, which is later strained; the liquid is applied with a cotton ball where needed. The leaves also can be included.

TO HARVEST: Gently pull the entire plant from the ground and use the stalk.

Plantain
(Plantago officinalis; P. lanceolata)

TYPE: perennial

HEIGHT: 6 to 18 inches

SMELL: not noticeable

COLOR: dark green leaves, brown seeds on tall
stalks, barely noticeable flowers

HABIT: Plantain is considered a weed all over
the world; also called Englishman's foot, it
spreads rapidly and can be found in wastelands,
driveways, yards, and parks. Plantain grows
very low to the ground and has small, wiry
leaves that form a rosette, though in rich soil
its leaves will grow wide and broad and its stalk
will be up to 18 inches tall. "Plantain" is also the
name of a tree which produces fruits similar to
a banana; this is an entirely different plant. The
herb plantain produces no fruit that we would
recognize; instead, it is a low-growing weed
that is easy to overlook and that unfortunately is
often pulled out of yards or mowed over.

EDIBLE: Yes, the young leaves in early spring are
edible, though they are rather tough and stringy.
The seeds are edible and very fibrous.

MEDICINE: Plantain is valuable in many ways. It is a
drawing herb, meaning it literally pulls things up
through the skin, making it ideal for bee stings.
If I chew a small leaf and place it on the sting,

one

I'll feel the leaf growing hot. I replace it with another chewed leaf, then another. After using about twenty leaves, the sting is gone. (Caution: make sure there is no life-threatening allergy first; this method is for symptomatic relief only.) Plantain is a great addition to a first aid ointment as it will heal wounds. The seeds are a good source of fiber and can be used to ease symptoms of diarrhea and support digestive health.

TO HARVEST: Pull each leaf individually from the center of the rosette; you'll notice it is very stringy. To harvest the seeds, strip them from the stalk and sprinkle them on oatmeal or other foods.

Pleurisy Root
(Asclepias tuberosa)

TYPE: perennial

HEIGHT: 12 to 36 inches

SMELL: not noticeable

COLOR: brilliant orange flowers atop dark green leaves and stalks

HABIT: Pleurisy root, also called butterfly weed, is related to milkweed; both are common pasture and meadow herbs, though some consider them unhealthy for livestock. Pleurisy root is listed on the United Plant Savers "to-watch" list, indicating that it is potentially in need of preservation in the wild. Once it is established in a garden, it self-seeds and replenishes itself easily. This herb grows upright but tends to lean, and its branches will sag and fall over to the side, sometimes breaking.

EDIBLE: No, though it is not poisonous either. However, farmers consider it poisonous to livestock.

MEDICINE: Pleurisy root is valued for its root as a lung remedy. It is traditionally used to ease both wet and dry coughs, lung spasms, and bronchial congestion. Many herbalists use it for cough, asthma, congestion, colds and flu, and other acute conditions.

TO HARVEST: Dig the root and harvest the entire plant; wash the roots thoroughly with a hose, then chop the root and make an alcohol tincture.

Red Clover
(Trifolium pratense)

TYPE: perennial

HEIGHT: 4 to 16 inches

SMELL: sweet, fragrant, honey-like

COLOR: pink or red blossoms, green leaves

HABIT: Red clover can be a ground cover or it can sprout up as a single wildflowering plant with tall stalks.

EDIBLE: Yes, the blossoms are edible and are good sprinkled in salads or brewed into tea.

MEDICINE: High in calcium, red clover is a good herb to include in mineral-rich infusions; it is vulnerary, meaning it is a good addition to first aid ointments, and as an emollient it is soothing and cooling to the skin. Red clover (as opposed to white clover) contains phytoestrogens and is used to support women's hormone balance, especially through menopause.

TO HARVEST: With your fingers, snip the entire flower head, including the blossom and top leaves.

St. John's Wort
(Hypericum perforatum)

TYPE: perennial

HEIGHT: 12 to 36 inches

SMELL: not noticeable

COLOR: dark green leaves; flowers are bright yellow
with tiny black or red dots

HABIT: Though St. John's wort can be considered an
invasive weed, I list it here as an herb to cultivate
or allow to grow wild because it is so useful
medicinally. St. John's wort grows in meadows,
fields, roadsides, woodland edges, and gardens.
It is an upright plant that often branches and is
rather see-through, meaning it is a sparse plant
and not full and bushy. It can be easy to overlook
if it is not in flower.

EDIBLE: St. John's wort leaves, flowers, and seeds
are edible in teas and sprinkled in salads, though
it is not considered a "food" herb and farmers
consider it poisonous to cattle.

MEDICINE: St. John's wort is a well-regarded medicine, especially in Europe, where it is marketed to treat mild to moderate depression. Traditional use holds that St. John's wort is a gladdening herb that eases anxiety, relieves sadness (especially seasonal blues) and treats depression. It should not be taken with other pharmaceutical antidepressants because it can escalate the amount of serotonin in the body to dangerous levels. On its own, St. John's wort is a safe alternative to antidepressants. Topically, this herb is useful in first aid ointments and salves to heal wounds; it produces a reddish-tinged oil or tincture due to oil glands located in its flowers and leaves that contain hypericin, a red-colored chemical.

TO HARVEST: Snip off the stalks near the base or near an "elbow" where a stem branches. Turn the stem upside down and strip the leaves and flowers in one stroke. Collect them in a bag. You'll notice your fingers will be stained red; this is normal. Use the leaves and flowers immediately by infusing them in oil or alcohol.

Violet
(Viola odorata)

TYPE: perennial

HEIGHT: 6 to 8 inches

SMELL: lightly fragrant

COLOR: dark green or purple leaves; light purple, pink, or white flowers

HABIT: Violets grow in small mounds, often forming a ground cover. They enjoy shady and moist places and will flourish if the air is cool and the water around them is clean and clear. The young leaves are soft and succulent and make a good food, and the flowers can be harvested easily by children, who enjoy popping the sweet, colorful blossoms into their mouths. Violets often appear in the spring and are spent by late summer; enjoy them early.

EDIBLE: Yes, both the leaf and the flower.

MEDICINE: Violets have many uses; similar to self-heal or heal-all, they support the work of other herbs. Use violet leaf and flower for respiratory support in cough syrups for dry coughs, and use the flower as an eye wash or rinse. Topically they are an excellent vulnerary to include in first aid ointments.

TO HARVEST: Snip fresh, small leaves with your fingers, and harvest flowers individually.

Yellow Dock/Burdock
(Rumex crispus / Arctium lappa)

TYPE: biennial

HEIGHT: 4 to 12 feet

SMELL: not noticeable

COLOR: Yellow dock leaves are dark green in summer and quickly tend toward yellow and brown, with brown flowers and seeds; burdock leaves are gray-green, and the seeds are brown.

HABIT: Both put up tall stalks with a flower that easily goes unnoticed and prolific seeds.

EDIBLE: Yes, burdock root is considered a vegetable in Eastern cuisine, being sautéed or boiled.

MEDICINE: Both plants are valued for their roots and seeds. Dock species (including yellow dock, granny dock, and curly dock) are traditionally used to support the body when it needs iron (for example, with anemia or loss of blood). Burdock is considered a hepatic herb, supporting the liver's ability to metabolize waste products. Both are traditionally used to "cleanse" the blood and liver. Use the roots and seeds for medicine and the seeds for fabric dye.

TO HARVEST: The roots are incredibly steadfast and require a lot of work to extract. Dig them up when the ground is wet and soft. Clean them well, chop them, and tincture them in vinegar, which is an excellent menstruum for pulling the minerals from the roots.

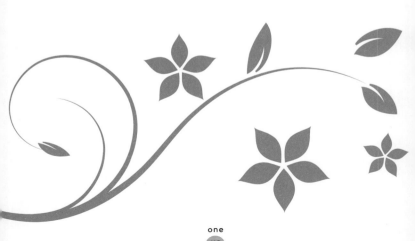

Herbs to Avoid for Your Garden's Sanity

Some herbs spread naturally and will quickly take over your garden. Each year is different; one year I had an explosion of wild geranium; one year it was Queen Anne's lace, and one year I had more lemon balm than I knew what to do with. Even the really wonderful and highly useful herbs will tend to spread if not kept in check: nettle, catnip, and anise hyssop are notorious spreaders.

But as many headaches as you might get from these herbs, and as many little pots you may use to dig up repeat offenders and offer them to friends, the following list contains herbs that you really never want to plant because your entire garden will be at risk for years to come. Be sure to remove these at every opportunity to ensure they never get rooted in your garden:

ground ivy · morning glory · mugwort ·
peppermint · sorrel · tansy · wild geranium

Herbal Properties

Now that you have a basic understanding of the forty main herbs that we're covering in the book, you may still be wondering which you would most like to plant and work with. The following chart should help you decide. It covers the properties of a plant—what a plant does in the body and why you'll find it useful medicinally. For instance, lavender is often used to help someone fall asleep; you'll find it in the chart under "sedative."

Refer to this chart as you decide which herbs you'd like to grow. For example, if you want to make a first aid salve, you'll want to plant herbs that are vulnerary because these herbs heal wounds.

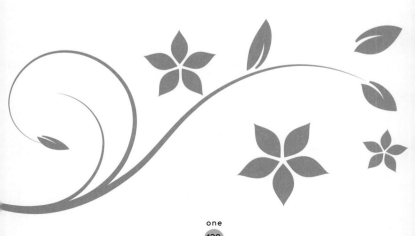

HERBAL PROPERTIES CHART

PROPERTIES	HERBS
ANALGESIC (RELIEVES PAIN)	CANNABIS DANDELION LAVENDER ST. JOHN'S WORT TURMERIC
ANTIMICROBIAL (CAN FIGHT OR KILL PATHOGENS)	ANISE HYSSOP CALENDULA CATNIP CHAMOMILE ELDERBERRY FENNEL GARLIC GINGER LAVENDER LEMON BALM OREGANO PLEURISY ROOT ROSEMARY SAGE SPEARMINT THYME YARROW
AROMATIC (HIGHLY FRAGRANT)	ANGELICA ANISE HYSSOP CATNIP CHAMOMILE FENNEL LAVENDER LEMON BALM ROSE ROSEMARY SAGE SPEARMINT

PROPERTIES	HERBS
ASTRINGENT (DRYING)	ROSEMARY SAGE YARROW
BITTER (OFTEN SUPPORTS DIGESTION)	CALENDULA CHAMOMILE DANDELION HOPS MOTHERWORT TURMERIC YARROW YELLOW DOCK
CARMINATIVE (STOMACH SOOTHER)	ANGELICA ANISE HYSSOP CATNIP CHAMOMILE FENNEL GINGER LAVENDER SPEARMINT
COUGH SUPPRESSANT	ANISE HYSSOP ELDERBERRY ELECAMPANE MALLOW PLEURISY ROOT VIOLET
DEMULCENT (SOOTHING AND COOLING, INTERNAL USE)	FENNEL HIBISCUS HOLY BASIL LEMON BALM MALLOW NETTLE PLANTAIN RED CLOVER SELF-HEAL VIOLET

PROPERTIES	HERBS
EMOLLIENT (SOOTHING AND COOLING, EXTERNAL USE)	BLACK CUMIN BORAGE CALENDULA ELDERBERRY FLOWER HOLY BASIL JEWELWEED LAVENDER LEMON BALM MALLOW PLANTAIN ROSE RED CLOVER SELF-HEAL ST. JOHN'S WORT VIOLET
EXPECTORANT (SUPPORTS RELEASE OF PHLEGM)	ANGELICA ANISE HYSSOP CATNIP ELDERBERRY FENNEL GARLIC GINGER OREGANO PLEURISY ROOT THYME
GALACTAGOGUE (INCREASES BREASTMILK)	ANGELICA FENNEL NETTLE RED CLOVER
HEART TONIC	BORAGE GARLIC HIBISCUS HOLY BASIL MOTHERWORT ROSE

PROPERTIES	HERBS
NERVINE TONIC	BORAGE
	CANNABIS
	CATNIP
	CHAMOMILE
	HOLY BASIL
	LAVENDER
	LEMON BALM
	MOTHERWORT
	NETTLE
	ROSE
	ST. JOHN'S WORT
	VALERIAN
SEDATIVE (SUPPORTS SLEEP)	CATNIP
	CHAMOMILE
	HOPS
	LAVENDER
	VALERIAN

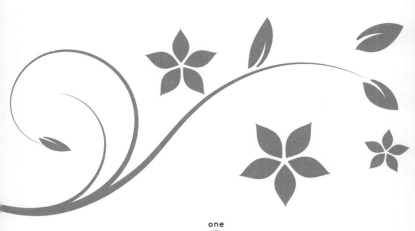

PROPERTIES

VULNERARY
(WOUND HEALING)

HERBS

ANISE HYSSOP
BLACK CUMIN
BORAGE
CALENDULA
CATNIP
DANDELION
ELDERBERRY LEAF & FLOWER
JEWELWEED
LAVENDER
LEMON BALM
MALLOW
OREGANO
PLANTAIN
RED CLOVER
ROSE
ROSEMARY
SAGE
SELF-HEAL
SPEARMINT
ST. JOHN'S WORT
THYME
VALERIAN
VIOLET
YARROW

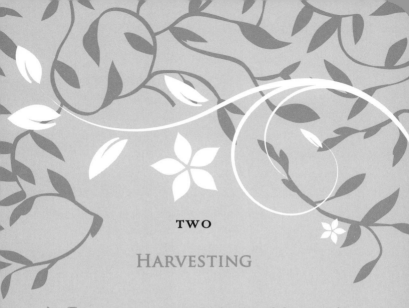

TWO

HARVESTING

N ow it's time to reap the bounty of the season's energy. The herbs and trees are bursting with flowers, leaves, berries and fruit, stalks, seeds, and roots that may be used as food and medicine. It's easy to snap off a berry here and there to enjoy, but if you're making a batch of remedies for yourself, your family, or your community, there are sustainable and effective ways to harvest that will make your remedies more potent and also keep your plants happy, too.

Let's start with a couple of philosophies that are good to follow when harvesting.

Permission and Gratitude

If you're accustomed to working with plants, you've probably come to realize that they possess a certain individuality—a certain personality or "being" of their own. Having worked with plants for several decades, learning that plants are entities and have their own energy has been a key lesson for me. Long ago I began asking a plant if it was willing to be harvested for a particular remedy. At first I asked out loud, speaking to the plant, and being someone who grew up in a society that laughed at such notions, I felt silly. I couldn't shake the strange feeling, so I went inward, asking in my mind, and it felt just fine. It was my energy speaking to the plant's energy, and it worked for me. Many herbalists speak and sing to their plants—such as at Findhorn Foundation in Scotland— but I find I'm a much more solitary and quiet herbalist who connects with plants in my mind and my heart. However you ask for permission, just connect and listen.

Gratitude is another lesson. Appreciating your harvest and your experience with plants can only be good. There are several ways to do this:

- Say thank you. Say it aloud or in your head. Mean it.

- Offer something in exchange. Sprinkle dried tobacco, dried calendula, bits of your hair, seeds from a packet of new plants ... however you choose to honor the gift of the plant is worthwhile.

- Teach others and share your gratitude.

Wildcrafting

Before we jump into the beautiful garden you've been tending, let's talk about wildcrafting. This is the art of harvesting plants that grow wild—you didn't plant them or tend them. Instead, they are growing wild and are full of vitamins, minerals, flavors, and medicine that you can enjoy and include in your remedies.

Learn all you can about these wild plants, especially as they are different in each region of the world. Find a good plant identification book specific to your region and go on walks with local herbalists to learn what grows around you. Explore your nearby woods, creeks, ponds, and meadows, and you'll likely find an abundant source of free, potent, and effective medicinal herbs such as plantain, St. John's wort, or elderberry. When wildcrafting, be sure of a few things before you start:

- Be certain the area has not been sprayed with herbicides or pesticides. These chemicals will reside in the plants and in the soil and can make you sick.

- Obtain permission to harvest, especially if you are on someone else's property.

- Observe the 1:10 rule; don't harvest more than one in every ten plants you see. For instance, if you come across a scattering of St. John's wort, don't collect them all. Don't even collect half. Harvest at most one in every ten, and then only harvest what you need. Many habitats and populations are at risk; this is especially true of herbs whose roots are harvested. If harvesting roots, try to replant some of them or learn if spreading the plant's seeds will help regenerate the population.

- Consult United Plant Savers. This nonprofit organization is dedicated to protecting and preserving wild medicinal herbs. They provide lists of herbs that are endangered or at risk of becoming endangered due to overharvesting, habitat loss, pollution, grazing, and the rampant building of houses, subdivisions, and parking lots. Consider supporting the herbal UPS, and follow their recommendations for harvesting at-risk plants.

- Wear protective clothing, and be prepared for weather changes. Be smart about being out in the wild, and don't put yourself at risk.

- Remember that wild plants aren't necessarily hundreds of miles in the deep interior; they can be right next to your home or growing along the edge of your fence. Weeds are wild, free, abundant, and effective.

Harvesting by the Moon

The moon has a profound effect on both nature and humanity; the moon controls the tides of all the oceans on Earth, and it is said that a full moon brings out emotions and can control the tenor of our relationships. More babies are born on full moons, more crimes happen on full moons, and generally we feel more social on full moons; our emotions rise to the surface, out of the depths of ourselves, and we feel full of energy. Similarly, the full moon draws up the energy of plants. Flowers that are of a normal energy in mid-month are traditionally seen to possess a stronger medicinal potency on a full moon.

Harvest your flowers, leaves, and seeds on a full moon, but wait until a new moon to harvest the roots, as this is when the moon's influence is weakest and the energy of the plant is comfortably down in the earth.

Does this mean you need to go out at midnight to harvest the aerial parts of the plant? Not necessarily, though many herbalists like to do this as it is beautiful to be in the garden at night under the light of a full moon. Harvesting lunar herbs—such as the artemesias, which are silvery and reflective—can be a ceremonial experience that can add an extra dimension of fun and meaning to your remedies.

Harvesting Throughout the Season

Experiment with the many creative ways to harvest herbs throughout the growing season. Some plants, such as nettles and lemon balm, can be harvested when they reach their succulent peak and then left to grow more throughout the season. Later, toward fall, they have grown enough to be harvested again. Definitely take advantage of these opportunities and learn to watch for the signs that a plant can be harvested twice—generally if it regrows after the first harvest, is a perennial, and doesn't get too leggy the second time around. If you plan to re-harvest a plant, be sure to provide it with extra mulch or food so that it is prepared to offer new growth.

Also consider the time of the season as a guide for harvesting the aerial parts (above-ground parts such as flowers, leaves, stalks, and seeds) or the underground parts. In the beginning of the season, especially along the East Coast, the leaves and flowers receive all the plant's attention, growing fat, lush, and juicy. This isn't the time to harvest roots, which are surrendering their energy to the above-ground parts. Later in the fall, after the leaves have browned or fallen and the flowers have turned to seed—and even after the seeds have blown or fallen—then it will be time for the roots to claim their part of the plant's energy. The roots will begin to stockpile sugars in preparation for the winter and will finally be at their best for medicine.

TIP 4

Baskets and Bags

Instead of keeping your gathering equipment out-side, find a place just inside your door to keep it, and train yourself to return your baskets and bags to their spot when you're finished. Hanging baskets on hooks from a rafter or on the wall is a great way to show off a pretty and functional item.

Harvesting Flowers and Leaves

If you have a love for herbs, you'll likely spend your spring and summer harvesting succulent young violet leaves to eat in your salad, velvety mallow leaves to tuck into fairy beds, or bright green lemon balm leaves to make into medicinal syrups and tinctures. You'll pick feathery yarrow leaves and strip the soft bits from the stem right onto your cutting board. You'll snap off entire leaf sets from elder bushes, and you'll gather flowers of every color you can imagine: creamy-white yarrow, lilac-colored sage, crimson bee balm, and sunshine-infused calendula petals. When harvesting, follow these tips to get the most from the leaves and flowers:

- Consider the phase of the moon, and harvest above-ground (aerial) parts such as leaves, flowers, and seeds on the full moon, when the energy is pulling upward from the earth. The energy from the plants will be in the above-ground parts, whereas at the new moon the energy will be underground.

- The best time to harvest, especially on hot days, is mid-morning. Wait until the dew has evaporated from the leaves and they are fairly dry, but don't wait too long because the midday sun will wilt the plants and weaken them. Dusk is also a good time to harvest, but mosquitoes can be troublesome.

- When harvesting from plants with larger leaves, such as plantain, elder, mallow, and anise hyssop, snip the leaves one by one. With smaller leaves, instead of harvesting leaf by leaf, snip off an entire branch or stalk and then strip the leaves in one fluid motion. For some plants, such as cleavers and wild yarrow, harvest the entire aerial (above-ground) plant. Chop cleavers as-is; strip yarrow leaves from the stalk. For other plants, such as catnip and peppermint, snip off a branch, leaving the rest of the plant to continue to grow.

Harvesting with fingers or a pair of small shears or snippers is usually appropriate; for some plants, though, you'll need an assortment of tools to get the job done. Nettles, for instance, require advanced planning and appropriate gear.

Harvesting Nettle

Nettle requires a little forethought when harvesting because each of the thousands of needles rests atop a sac filled with histamine and stinging formic acid. Don't worry too much about being stung; the sting will last from twenty minutes to a few hours, but it's not life-threatening and is generally no more than a nuisance. If it brushes against your skin, apply some first aid ointment or salve (see chapter 3) or break open a stalk of jewelweed and rub the juice on the skin. These will soothe the rash and the sting will subside.

While harvesting, wear protective gear; prepare lightweight gloves, kitchen tongs, scissors, a large paper grocery bag or a bucket with a handle, and a wide bowl. Put on the gloves, open the grocery bag or place the bucket beside you, and place the tongs in one hand and the scissors in the other. Using the tongs, hold the stalk you wish to cut and snip at the base of the stalk with the scissors, near the ground. Place the stalk into the bag or bucket, angling the base of the stalk in first so that the leaves or flowers are sticking out. Repeat until you have all the stalks you want.

Then, inside at the kitchen counter or outside on the picnic table, hold one stalk with the tongs and use the scissors to snip off all the leaves, one by one, letting them drop into the wide bowl. Compost the stalks or make a tea with them. If you've harvested full, lush, young leaves, you can move these from the bowl to a food processor; add olive oil and salt to make pesto or add cream cheese to make a dip.

If the leaves are older, smaller, and tougher, they will probably be best as a tea. Snip them into a large pot filled with water, along with the stalks, and bring to just under a boil. Steep for twelve to fifteen minutes. It's ready to drink at this point, but for a stronger and more mineral-rich infusion, put the lid on the pot and allow it to steep on very low heat for several hours or turn the heat off and allow it to sit, covered, overnight. Strain the solids out in the morning (if you didn't include stalks, these solids can be placed in the food processor and made into a dip). Reheat if desired and store the tea in a thermos to drink throughout the day or place in the refrigerator for iced tea.

TIP 5

Tools versus Fingers

Use snippers, scissors, and shovels where appropriate, but don't forget the value of your own fingers for harvesting. Being able to touch a plant can add to the enjoyment of working in nature. When possible, snip leaves and flowers with your fingers for a more direct experience.

Harvesting Seeds

Seeds are a plant's promise, the universe's babies, the repositories of all that has come and all that will be. Seeds are a bank from which lifetimes of deposits have been made and from which we can withdraw wisdom, beauty, and nourishment. Seeds have momentum and mobility of their own—clinging onto birds and dogs and rabbits to travel to other places or puffing themselves up to float on the waters of a creek, river, or ocean. Think of the burdock seeds attaching themselves to your socks when you walk or of a coconut flipping itself from its tall perch onto the rollicking waves beneath it. Seeds have life.

They also offer nutrition—minerals, vitamins, fiber, and omega fatty acids that make them prime nourishment for human bodies and minds. Nettle seeds are being studied for their protection of the prostate, milk thistle seeds protect our livers, and chia seeds are high in protein. Many seeds, such as mallow seeds, are high in protein and potassium; fennel seeds not only taste good but are excellent for stomach upset and will help the digestive system work properly. Cilantro seeds are called coriander, and these, along with caraway seeds, aid digestion. White pepper is the seed of the black pepper with the surrounding fruit stripped away; it is a culinary spice. Vitex berries, commonly called chaste tree, are harvested at the seed stage, when they can be easily stripped from the branch and collected for tincturing.

I've generally found two methods for harvesting seeds: in the first, simply hold a large paper bag beneath a branch or stem and strip the seeds into it with your fingers. This works well for vitex. In the second, use the fingers to harvest the entire seed head. This works well for fennel and angelica. When tincturing it is not necessary to remove every little bit of stem attached to the seed; if you're using the seeds for culinary purposes, remove as much as you can.

Harvesting Roots

Unlike seeds, which are the plant's way to spread itself and promise new and different life, a plant's roots are its way to center itself and promise its own continuation. After a sunny growing season, a perennial plant will let its upper parts die back, and it will focus its energy by literally sending sugars and other nourishment down into the ground to its roots, where it will feed on this energy source all winter. From this energy bank, it will draw what it needs to sprout up again in the spring. Many roots have vitamin A, such as sweet potatoes, which is great for our eyes and skin, as well as the immune system. Many are used medicinally, such as pleurisy root for its expectorant properties, useful for bronchial infections, or valerian root for its antispasmodic properties and its sedative action.

When harvesting roots, choose a new moon if possible, and do the harvest in the fall after the aerial parts have died back. Dig with a garden spade—it's shaped like a spading shovel but has tines like a pitchfork. It may be called a digging spade, a spading shovel, or a spading fork. These are easier than shovels because they allow dirt to move through the tines and it's not as heavy to lift or hard on the back. Start by pushing the spade into the ground about six inches from the center of the plant, at about a 45-degree angle toward the root. Push in, lift and wiggle the fork a bit, then pull out and move to your right or left, working your way around the plant in a circle. Push in, lift, pull out, move. Do this until you've completed a circle around the plant. For large plants such as pleurisy root, this is the only way to get the plant out of the ground, as it needs to be worked from all directions. Smaller plants such as wild geranium can be maneuvered out with a hand trowel.

• EXERCISE 3 •
Harvesting Valerian

Valerian is a tall, fragrant herb, valuable as an anti-inflammatory and pain reliever (analgesic). It is also valued as a
sedative. Harvest both its flowers and root to infuse them
into olive oil for a muscle rub or into grain alcohol for a
tincture. To harvest its root:

STEP 1: Chop off the stalk a few inches above the
   ground so you can access the center of the plant.

STEP 2: Stand next to the plant and, using your boot,
   press the spading fork into the ground at an angle.
   Press down so the plant lifts up slightly, then pull
   out.

STEP 3: Move around the plant in a circle, pushing in,
   lifting, and pulling out.

STEP 4: Pulling on the bottom of the stalk, lift the
   entire plant from the ground. Shake as much dirt
   off as you can (smack the roots against a piece of
   wood or fence). You want the dirt to stay in the
   garden.

STEP 5: Using a garden hose, spray the roots carefully.
   Valerian roots look like spaghetti. Once all the

dirt has been sprayed away and the roots are clean, place the entire chunk on a cutting board, preferably on a picnic table.

STEP 6: Using a sharp knife or a hatchet, separate the roots from the top of the mass. You won't need the parts at the top, just the juicy white roots. Chop them into half-inch or one-inch pieces. You may rinse them again in a colander if you wish.

STEP 7: Place the roots in a glass canning jar and cover with the menstruum (liquid) of your choice. Generally I use vodka or Everclear for tinctures.

Fresh versus Dried

For most herbal remedies, use fresh plant material—fresh leaves, flowers, and roots. Fresh ingredients make the best remedies. Salves made with fresh plant material boast richer colors: dark green yarrow ointments, dark yellow and orange calendula salves. Tinctures turn a bright red with fresh St. John's wort or a bright purple with fresh violet flowers. (You can obtain similar results with dried plant material by simmering the herbs longer in olive oil.)

Dried ingredients shine when making teas. As well, tisanes, infusions, and decoctions are at their best when made from properly dried leaves and flowers. Dried roots require a much longer steeping time when making teas; this is called making a decoction.

Label Properly

After you harvest, especially if you're using fresh plants, you'll need to immediately process your herbs. If you're making tinctures, the first step is to place the cleaned, chopped herbs into a glass canning jar and add the alcohol. This canning jar will sit in your pantry or cabinet for weeks if not months, therefore labeling this canning jar is important. From this jar you'll strain and decant the tincture and pour the liquid into smaller bottles for individual use. Learning to label the glass canning jar is a priority. This is also true when you're making vinegar tinctures, topical oils (such as infused olive oil that will be included in salves, ointments, or massage blends), and more. The herbs will infuse in the alcohol, vinegar, and oil in the glass canning jar, and this part of the process requires a certain amount of care.

You'll want to know what is in your jars in a few weeks; opening your pantry and seeing an unlabeled half-gallon jar sitting among a half-dozen other jars can be disappointing. Sticky labels will fall off the sides of jars quickly, tape will dry or rot, and ink on paper will fade. Label the jar twice—once directly on the lid using a permanent marker and once on the side by taping a paper label to the jar with strong packaging tape. Include this information on the label:

- the date
- the herbs inside
- the liquid inside
- if you're going to start selling your creations, include a batch number and keep this information in a file

Refer to the following samples to create your own labels.

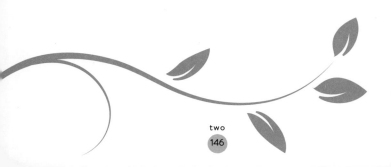

Yarrow Leaf Tincture

in alcohol (vodka)
no water added

harvested and bottled June 21, 2020

 Batch #0621

 Lemon Balm & Rose Tincture

Herb 1: Lemon Balm Leaf · Source: garden, fresh
Herb 2: Rose Petal · Source: store, dried
(lot #125 from Local Apothecary Inc.)
Menstruum: vodka 75% · glycerine 25%

bottled June 21, 2020 · Batch #0621

BASIC LABEL (TOP), DETAILED LABEL (BOTTOM)

Small Jars, Small Batches

Use small jars if you are just starting out. Even a very small garden plot can produce volumes of herbs—great quantities of green foliage and huge roots that erupt from the ground with your shovel. You may have mountains of herbs to work with from just a few plants—for instance, one can harvest bags and bags of leaves from just a couple of lemon balm plants—and instead of purchasing twenty to forty half-gallon canning jars and spending a fortune on vodka, I would suggest using this abundance of herbal material in creative ways. Instead of making a half-dozen jars of, say, lemon balm tincture, you could:

- make quantities of lemon balm tea and pour some of it into ice cube trays to freeze
- infuse a variety of oils with the leaves to make a lotion or massage oils
- hang some of it to dry for later use
- place some of it in jars with oil for salves
- chop some of it into a pot with honey and make infused honey
- make a giant pot of lemon balm "tea" and pour it in a hot, freshly drawn bath for soaking in

- *and* place a small portion of it in jars with vodka or brandy for tinctures

You may have enough lemon balm (or spearmint or lavender or catnip) to experiment broadly and make all of these in one season.

The point is, you could easily let yourself get carried away with tincture bottles, enjoying the glint of glass and the organized look of neat rows of jars on your shelf. And if you're using or selling these tinctures, this is great. But if you're making them for your family or even as gifts, it's easy to have way too much, especially of something you might eventually realize that you aren't really going to use that much of—such as violet flower tincture. If you end up with a half-gallon of violet flower tincture, you may smile later and wonder what you had planned to do with it all. Tinctures, after all, are given by the ¼ teaspoon, with about 25 drops being a dose, and you will be taking violet flower tincture until you are 100 years old. (In the next chapter you'll find a liquid extracts chart that will be helpful for when you're choosing the liquids in which you will infuse the herbs … more on that later.)

So, my recommendation is to begin with small jars for tinctures—perhaps pint jars—when you're starting out, and allow yourself to get creative by making other worthy remedies, too. I also recommend purchasing new pint jars for this purpose instead of reusing bottles or jars from your kitchen. This is partly to keep things uniform and partly to guard against spoilage and spilling. It's also easier to keep your labels straight and, in my experience, uniformly sized jars are easier to organize and use.

How to Dry Herbs

Using herbs fresh is the best method for oils, salves, and tinctures, but dried herbs make the best teas. There are several ways to dry herbs:

DEHYDRATOR: An electric dehydrator is a great choice for small things like rose petals; they'll curl up crisp and retain their color and heavenly smell. Downside: it uses electricity, and it is yet another appliance to store in your home. The best herbs for a dehydrator are rose petals, lemon balm leaves, violet flowers, calendula flowers, fennel fronds, rosehips, and elderberries.

NEWSPRINT: For a simple method, spread a few layers of newspaper on the floor or on a table where it won't be trampled or blown by a breeze. An attic is an ideal place for this. Spread the stalks or branches of your herbs in single layers; don't strip the leaves off until they are crisp-dry.

HANGING IN PAPER BAGS: While bunches of herbs hung along the rafters of the kitchen look beautiful and charming, they aren't really potent and are more for looks than for use. However, hanging has its place, especially if you hang the herbs from a nail or hook and then encase them in a brown paper bag. This retains the color and also catches bits of flower or leaf that may fall from the stalk during the drying process. When the plant is dry, simply remove the plant, shake it inside the bag, and strip the leaves from the stalk directly into the bag.

SCREENS: An old screen from a door or window is a great vehicle for drying herbs. See exercise 4 for instructions to help you easily dry your herbs on screens.

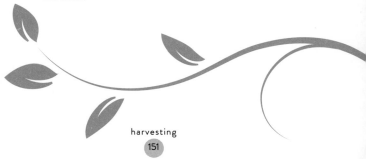

harvesting

TIP 6

Using Dehydrators

When you've harvested juicy herbs with a high water content, dry them on a screen or newsprint first. Once they've wilted, move them to a food dehydrator to get them fully dry.

• EXERCISE 4 •
Screen Drying

Get creative with this process: place the screen across two sawhorses, in the backseat of a warm car, or—my favorite—affixed to the top of a staircase between the railing and the wall. Warm air rises up the stairs and dries the herbs on its way. Many herbalists like warm, drafty attics: they are dry and generally dark, two key elements in drying herbs while maintaining their potency.

STEP 1: **Position the Screen.** Choose a place that is fairly dark and well-ventilated but not windy. Avoid places that are balmy or moist, such as kitchens. Even though the top of the refrigerator is warm, it's too wet and greasy, and your herbs will not dry properly.

STEP 2: **Collect Your Herbs** (stalks of lemon balm, stalks of boneset, individual comfrey leaves, branches of mint, heads of elderflower, etc). Spread them out in a single layer on the screen.

STEP 3: **Wait a Few Weeks.** When the herbs are completely crisp, strip the dried leaves or flowers from their stalks into your waiting container. Now you can make your remedies or potpourri.

THREE

MAKING

Handcrafting is a skill, an art, a tradition. It's an experience of folk medicine on the deepest level, a way that our mothers and grandmothers, fathers and great-uncles preserved their harvests and enjoyed Mother Nature's bounty. To handcraft is to make herbal remedies from the leaves, flowers, seeds, stalks, and roots you've just collected and appreciate the value of those plants and feel grateful. To handcraft is to honor the connection between the plants and ourselves—to recognize the healing benefits from plants for our bodies and minds.

Herbs are the "people's pharmacy," the stock pantry for all our illnesses and needs, the little chapel in the woods for our heart's recovery. Herbs and trees are the medicine of the people, straight from the earth.

Best of all, it's fun to handcraft! Making medicine is a hands-on activity that gets better with practice and is always useful. Remedies aren't necessarily meant to be beautifully packaged and gleaming, ready to place on a sales shelf. Instead, herbal remedies are intended to support, to nourish, to heal; even the most humble little jar with a cork in it can be the needed balm for the soul.

Get Everyone Involved

Thanks to its simplicity, herbal medicine making can include everyone in the family, especially children. There are so many ways a child can be involved on medicine-making day: let your child pick the berries, snip off the leaves, shred leaves, pick flowers, or push in the shovel around a plant when digging roots. Let your child pour oil into a pot, draw water from the faucet, push the buttons on the blender, drop chopped leaves into a bowl. One of my fondest memories is making lotion with my daughter when she was young; by the end of the morning we were both covered in lotion, our hands, arms, and faces smeared with oils. Neither one of us could pick anything up because our hands were so slippery.

It's easy to turn a medicine-making day into a group experience; invite your neighbors—even those you think might not be interested. It may surprise you to find out they've been curious what you're doing and even waiting for an invitation. Invite children—yours and their friends, and welcome the diversions that come along with that (such as leaving medicine-making to go into the woods to build a fairy house or taking the honey you were about to use and making sandwiches).

Don't forget your grandparents, and if you don't have grandparents nearby, adopt some. The older generation may not feel the need to get their hands involved, but they may be happy to sit and talk while you work. They also may be excited to be the beneficiaries of your soaps, lotions, and hot teas.

Mornings are the best time to make remedies. Gather interested children and friends in the morning to harvest fresh herbs. Assign tasks such as assembling jars and lids or spreading plants out on a screen. If you've forgotten an ingredient, an early start allows you time to harvest or find it. Sometimes salves require additional time to cool and solidify, so a morning start ensures there's no rush. Regardless of what time of day you choose, be sure to allow plenty of time so the process is efficient and enjoyable.

Supplies on the Cheap

Making herbal remedies needn't be expensive. Aside from a few select ingredients (such as pure beeswax or olive oil), most ingredients and packaging materials can be found very inexpensively. Just make sure whatever container you use is clean and very dry before you pour your salve into it.

Reusing and repurposing packaging materials is a thrifty way to let handcrafting become part of your daily life. For instance, cleaned baby jars can become salve or ointment jars; newsprint can serve a second life as an herb-drying material; and cleaned bottles with cleaned lids can be put to use for syrups, honeys, and vinegars. Preparation and crafting supplies can be found cheaply, too; at your local thrift store, look for:

- a glass or enamel saucepan
- whisks
- long-handle spoons (wooden, preferably)
- cutting boards (avoid wood as they tend to splinter)
- small glass jars with lids
- ceramic pots with cork lids
- small spray bottles

- glass canning jars with lids
- bowls of all sizes
- scissors, tongs, ladles, and small sharp knives
- fabric, needle, and thread
- unused labels or decorative stickers
- Pyrex or glass measuring cups with pouring lips
- funnels of all shapes and sizes

Liquids to Use for Your Medicine-Making

The next thing to consider is liquids. Consuming herbs fresh from the garden means using them as food; to create a medicine with them, we generally extract their properties into a liquid. This creates a concentrate. There is a wide variety of liquids available to us for medicine-making; in the order of increasing strength, the most common are water, milk, honey, oil, vinegar, witch hazel and isoporopyl acohol, and grain alcohol.

Each of these liquids is a common household product: water can be tap water, though many prefer distilled; milk can be pasteurized or not and can also include nut and legume milks; try to purchase honey from a local beekeeper, and always be sure your honey has not been bleached, sugared, or diluted; oil is your preference—when making medicines I prefer a good quality olive oil (it need not be extra virgin olive oil if it will be used as a topical remedy), and here I provide a recipe using coconut oil; vinegar refers to apple cider vinegar, or ACV, with or without "the mother"; and witch hazel and isopropyl alcohol can be purchased at any pharmacy or health food store. The only thing that may be uncommon is grain alcohol; this must be purchased at a licensed facility such as a liquor store. See page 191 for a more complete description of using alcohol to make herbal tinctures.

To determine the best liquid for your project, refer to the following chart, which provides basic information on how to pair liquids with appropriate herbs, safety, shelf life, and strength of final product.

LIQUID EXTRACTS CHART

LIQUID	INSTRUCTION
WATER	THE SAFEST, WATER MAKES A TEA OR A RINSE. SHORT SHELF LIFE: USE WITHIN A DAY. DECOCTIONS AND INFUSIONS ARE STRONGEST WATER EXTRACTS. TAKE 1–3 CUPS DAILY.
MILK	SOFT PLANT PARTS SUCH AS FLOWER PETALS AND LEAVES INFUSE WELL INTO BOTH COW MILK AND NUT MILKS; CONSIDER ROSES IN MILK FOR PUDDING OR CHAMOMILE IN WARM MILK AT BEDTIME.

HONEY	INFUSE HERBS INTO WARM HONEY, STRAIN, AND USE AS-IS. ALSO STIR POWDERED HERBS INTO HONEY (ELECTUARY) OR MIX WITH ACV TO CREATE A SWEET-TART OXYMEL. EXPERIMENT WITH MILD OR LIGHT HONEYS (SUCH AS RED CLOVER) AS WELL AS STRONGER AND MORE ROBUST HONEYS (SUCH AS DARK BROWN BUCKWHEAT)— EACH WILL GIVE YOUR FINISHED PRODUCT A DISTINCT TASTE AND COLOR.
OIL	MOSTLY FOR EXTERNAL APPLICATIONS. INFUSE OLIVE OIL WITH HERBS, STRAIN, AND ADD BEESWAX TO MAKE A SALVE. TO MAKE MASSAGE OILS, INFUSE LIGHTER OILS SUCH AS SUNFLOWER, JOJOBA, OR SWEET ALMOND WITH HERBS, THEN STRAIN.
VINEGAR	ACV IS PREFERRED, BUT ALMOST ANY VINEGAR WILL EXTRACT CHEMICALS FROM HERBS. WARM THE VINEGAR FIRST AND LET SIT TWO WEEKS, THEN STRAIN.
WITCH HAZEL AND ISOPROPYL ALCOHOL	HERBS INFUSED INTO RUBBING ALCOHOL (ISOPROPYL) MAKE A LINIMENT. USE HERB-INFUSED WITCH HAZEL AS A TOPICAL ASTRINGENT FOR WEEPY SORES. INFUSE UP TO TWO WEEKS.
GRAIN ALCOHOL	SOFTER LIQUORS (BRANDY, WINE) ARE BEST FOR SOFT PLANT PARTS. HARDER LIQUORS (VODKA, EVERCLEAR, WHISKEY) WILL EXTRACT ROOTS AND BARKS. THESE HAVE THE LONGEST SHELF LIFE OF ALL THE LIQUIDS—POTENTIALLY YEARS. STRONGEST EXTRACTS: TAKE 25 DROPS THREE TIMES DAILY (ON AVERAGE).

making

Decide What Remedy You Will Make

Now that you've chosen your herbs, it's time to choose a remedy. Do you want a topical remedy for the skin? A delicious remedy such as a tea or an oxymel? (These will both be covered in this section.) Or perhaps you want to create a medicine that is taken in small doses for common illnesses? Each of these is possible with the herbs on the provided lists. Options you can choose from—and that we'll be covering here—include brewing teas using a variety of methods; making remedies for the skin such as beeswax salves, coconut oil salves, lotion, face cream, spritzers, and baths; and remedies for internal use such as tinctures using alcohol or vinegar and remedies using honey. Because tea is the safest, easiest, and most versatile, let's start with learning to brew tea.

Brewing Delicious and Healing Tea

Teas, or herbal infusions, are the simplest and most enjoyable way to use the herbs you've grown and harvested. I use the term "tea" loosely, referring to true tea (with the *Camellia sinensis* plant) as well as herbal infusions and decoctions. However you make them, water-based plant extracts are delicious, fortifying, nutritious, medicinal, and great social opportunities because they are perfect for sharing with someone you love.

Teas are versatile: they can be enjoyed hot, cold, or room temperature. They can be sweet or tangy. They can be heavy and rich, like a chai, or light and summery, using lemon balm or roses. Teas can be medicinal and healing or they can simply be enjoyed. With a good thermos, they are portable and convenient because you can make a pot in the morning and keep it with you, ready to drink, all day long.

I highly recommend teas for all ages, especially children; plants offer so many benefits that surpass nutrition—they provide a connection to the natural world, especially if a child gets to harvest the plant in person. Plants are a source of beauty and can be a solace to a child facing anxiety or stress. The simple act of boiling water and brewing tea can be an introduction to the beauty of ritual and the value of ceremony. Drinking tea is also an opportunity to teach a child about different flavors—bold, rich, deep, lemony, bitter, tangy, minty, sweet, pungent, astringent, and floral.

Once you've made a tea, consider how you will use it. If you want to drink it, the following exercises will teach you how to brew teas and get the most enjoyment out of them. But there are many ways to use tea; see chapter 4 to discover a variety of ways to use tea in the kitchen, the house, and the yard.

There are a number of ways to make tea. Here we will explore three: brewing hot tea, making sun tea, and making iced tea.

• EXERCISE 5 •
Brewing Hot Tea

Only recently have I become a coffee drinker, so my foray into herbal teas began as it does for many: boiling a little water and pouring it over a tea bag into a cup. This is sufficient, but there is a lot more magic out there waiting for you if you're still in the bag-in-a-teacup days!

First, abandon the teabag, at least most of the time. If you have the option to brew loose-leaf herbs, please do. This process immerses both the herbs and your senses; by investing in a teapot that you like (a decent-sized glass or ceramic teapot that will hold at least four cups), you will avail yourself of creative and sensory options. Most tea bags are filled with "filings" or dregs, the bits that fall away from the cut herb in the manufacturing process. These are less tasty than coarsely chopped herbs that have been processed carefully; when you grow your own or purchase loose-leaf cut and dried herbs, you get better quality than what you purchase in most tea bags. Also, you now have the chance to collect a variety of herbs to add to this teapot.

To make a traditionally brewed tea, find a kettle and a teapot. Fill the kettle with water and set it on the stove on high heat. While it's heating, fill the teapot with the flowers and shredded leaves. If using fresh herbs, use a full handful (about a half cup) per cup of boiling water; if using dried herbs, use one teaspoon herbs per cup of boiling water.

Here are some blending suggestions:

> *Nourishing, bone-building blend:* nettle, self-heal, lemon balm
>
> *Digestive blend:* catnip, spearmint, fennel, ginger root
>
> *Stress support blend:* holy basil, nettle, hops, borage
>
> *Restful nighttime blend:* chamomile, catnip, rose petal, lavender

At the peak of summer, you'll be able to find abundant flowers and leaves with which to make a delicious tea: crimson-colored bee balm, pink red clover, golden calendula, purple violets, red-dotted St. John's wort, purple anise hyssop. Gather fennel, yarrow, elderflower, and spearmint. Snip lemon balm, catnip, lavender, sage, and holy basil leaves. Don't forget rose petals, and put on your gloves for nettle leaves.

Just as the water begins to boil, take the kettle off the heat and pour it over the herbs in the teapot. Put the lid on the teapot and let it sit, brewing, for eight to twelve minutes. For a stronger-tasting brew, and a beverage with the highest concentration of minerals, allow the tea to steep longer—for several hours or even overnight. This is called an infusion, and it is considered more medicinal than a tea or tisane. The lid captures the volatile (essential) oils that will evaporate in the heat. The heat will extract many more pigments and other chemicals from the herbs, making a brewed tea much darker in color and richer in flavor than a sun tea (see exercise 6). When you're ready, sweeten if desired and pour the tea through a strainer into tea cups or mugs, or into a thermos to keep it hot for hours. Compost the herbs.

TIP 7

Using a Thermos to Store Hot Tea

The beauty of brewing four cups of tea at once is that you can strain the tea from the teapot directly into a large thermos and keep it hot for hours. You no longer need to re-brew tea throughout the day, and you have ready access to fresh, hot, nutritious tea all day, which is especially nice in cold weather. For most medicinal teas, a daily dose is three to four cups, which makes a four-cup thermos perfect. Consider getting one that has a built-in drinking cup so that it is convenient to carry and drink throughout the day. Compost the herbs from the teapot, give it a rinse, and it's ready for the next day's brew.

Making Sun Tea

Gather your herbs and place them in a large glass jar, such as a two-gallon pickle jar often used at delis. Toss in all your flowers, then gently shred the leaves with your fingers and toss them in as well. Fill the jar with clean, cold water and place it in a sunny spot, such as on your porch or deck, where it won't get tipped over and where it will get full sun exposure. Place a lid on it or drape a cloth or tea towel over it to keep the bugs out. Let it sit in the full sun at least four hours and preferably all day; give the jar a swirl now and then to move the herbs around in the water.

Over the hours, the water will become colored by the pigments in the herbs and may turn a light red, pink, or pale green, and the flavor will be a mild and pleasant herbal flavor. To sweeten iced tea, either gently heat the tea in a saucepan to add honey or sugar, or avoid heating it and add apple juice as a sugar substitute. When you're ready, strain the herbs out and pour the tea into glasses; decorate the glasses with ice cubes you've made with flowers (see exercise 22) or add a small fresh sprig of lemon balm or lavender to each glass. This makes a mild-flavored tea that you can enjoy as-is or to which you can add ginger ale or soda, apple juice, or slices of fruit.

Making Iced Tea

To make delicious, colorful and tasty iced tea, use one of the previous methods and allow the tea to cool. Place the container in the refrigerator until it is chilled. Taste it occasionally, adding more water to dilute it if necessary. Sun tea makes a light-flavored tea that benefits from extra fruit juice or slices of fruit, while brewed hot tea makes a normal-flavored tea that benefits from extra sweetener, to which you can add lemonade or slices of lemon. Serve the iced tea in a glass container to which you add slices of fruit, whole flowers, or ice cubes (see exercise 22).

Dosage for Medicinal Teas

Generally, there are two dosages with herbal medicines: one for adults and one for children. Some herbalists use mathematical calculations based on age or weight, but I prefer a folk method that is relevant for most adults and kids of normal weight. It recommends:

- Adults: 2 to 3 cups of medicinal tea daily
- Children: ½ to 2 cups of medicinal tea daily

Very young children such as toddlers need less, and babies get tiny doses of tea by the dropperful (or, better yet, through the mother's milk). Doses of tinctures are quite different because they are made with grain alcohol and highly concentrated herbs, but teas, which are water-based, are taken by the cup. Use common sense when taking medicinal teas.

Remedies for the Skin

Herbal products for the skin are ideal ways to begin your journey into apothecary work. Skin products smell heavenly and are easy to apply; you don't need to worry about dosage or too many contraindications. Salves, ointments, and balms are all words for roughly the same product: they are fairly thick, slightly greasy, and stored in a small jar or tin. Lotion and cream are roughly the same; they are thinner, lightly greasy, and are stored in small jars or bottles with pumps. Each of these is based on infused oils and is meant to make our skin supple, moisturized, and youthful-feeling. We can also spritz our skin with scented sprays and immerse our bodies in healing water baths. There are so many ways to use herbs for the skin that many herbalists open skin-care and cosmetic businesses and never look back.

Here we will focus on some of the easiest remedies to make; these are fairly quick, inexpensive, and safe, and they use those wonderful herbs you've been harvesting.

• EXERCISE 8 •
Making Beeswax Salves

These are among my favorite remedies to make, as they are easy and fun and you can make a quantity fairly quickly to give as gifts (see chapter 4 for gift basket ideas). Here we will use beeswax, which is of higher quality and creates a better consistency than any other wax. Vegan herbalists can make coconut oil salves (see exercise 9). Be sure to purchase unbleached beeswax, ideally from your local beekeeper, and buy in blocks instead of beads or pearls, as these don't work as well.

Salves are meant to be slathered on the skin as moisturizing medicines; depending on the herbs you use in them, they can heal burns (lavender, St. John's wort, mallow, plantain), wounds (yarrow, mint, elder leaf, plantain, red clover, St. John's wort), eczema (calendula, black cumin), psoriasis (calendula, red clover, violet), and more. A first aid kit should have a good herbal salve in it that serves as an all-purpose ointment for boo-boos, bug bites, rashes, and lacerations. Be careful with punctures,

171

though, as bacteria can inhabit the deeper parts of the wound even though it may be healing on the top; for this reason, avoid comfrey leaf on punctures. You may have heard of "drawing" salves, an old-fashioned word for an herb that pulls things from the body. Plantain draws out splinters and is excellent to place on bee stings as it will pull the poison from the skin.

Determine if you will use essential oils; these are the volatile oils from plants that are aromatic and give a plant its scent. Distilled from the rest of the plant, the oils are highly concentrated and should not be consumed internally, but a few drops can be added to your salve. Adding essential oils will accomplish three things: it will give the salve a scent, it will act as a preservative to extend the shelf life of the salve, and it will function as an antibacterial agent, killing germs on contact and supporting the healing of a wound. Remember that because plants must be distilled into a concentrate, it takes a huge quantity of herbal material to yield a tiny bit of essential oil; therefore, use them sparingly and be aware of whether the oils you purchase were distilled from wild (and therefore vulnerable) populations of plants or from cultivated (and renewable) plants. Do not use hydrosols or flower waters in your salves because the water content is too high; with salves, you want to avoid moisture as much as possible.

Gather your utensils and line up your empty glass jars, placing their lids to the side. I usually start with three cups of oil (preferably olive but not safflower or sunflower), which will yield seven or eight two-ounce jars of salve. Harvest your fresh herbs and chop them coarsely; make sure they are not too wet and are in fact fairly dry. Some herbs, such as comfrey leaf, release a lot of moisture when they are chopped—lay them on some newsprint for a few hours to wilt a bit before placing them in your oil.

Next, determine the infusion method you will use: time or heat.

Time

This method lets the herbs steep at room temperature for about two weeks. An advantage is that you can include solar and lunar energies in the infusion, and you know the oil and the herbs haven't been cooked inappropriately. Disadvantage: you must wait. To use this method, place your chopped herbs in a glass canning jar, pour in the oil, lid and label the jar, and store it on a shelf. Shake it occasionally; when ready to use, strain the herbs out.

Heat

This method uses heat to extract the properties from the plants and accomplishes it in about twenty minutes to three hours. An advantage is its quick turnaround; a disadvantage is that you may overcook the herbs or burn them. To use this method, place your chopped herbs in a saucepan on the stove or, better yet, in a slow cooker. Pour in the oil and gently simmer on very low heat for up to three hours. Do not let it bubble or burn! When ready to use, strain the herbs out.

STEP 1: Chop your herbs and choose either the time method or the heat method; infuse your herbs into the oil. When the oil is ready, strain out your infused oil and pour it into a four-cup glass measuring cup with a pouring lip, filling it to the three-cup line.

STEP 2: On a cutting board, use a sharp paring knife to chop the beeswax into grape-sized chunks. Measure three-fourths cup of beeswax chunks with a measuring cup. Set aside.

STEP 3: Pour the infused oil into the saucepan and add the beeswax. Place the pan on low heat on the stovetop and slowly stir it while the beeswax melts.

STEP 4: Now things speed up. When the beeswax has all melted, carefully but quickly pour the oil from the hot saucepan into a glass measuring cup with a pouring lip (it can be the same one you used before). Then, carefully and quickly fill up each salve jar; I find it is easiest to pick up the salve jar and hold it in front of my face and pour from this height rather than leaving the jar on the table. It's less messy. Use caution holding hot glass jars.

STEP 5: If you're using essential oils, now is the time to drop 5 to 7 drops of oil into each salve jar. Immediately put the lids on and push the jars to the side so they can cool off and solidify. You'll notice that as they cool, they turn from dark to light starting at the bottom of the jar and moving upwards. Wait an hour or so, and when all the jars are completely cooled, tighten the lids and add the label to the side of the jar or to the lid. The shelf life is approximately one and a half years if stored in a cool location such as a pantry or cabinet.

TIP 8

❋

Making Salves: Keep It Dry

The number one tip to remember when making salves is to keep everything dry! The leaves or herbs you're using should be wilted or fairly dry, not juicy. The spoons, strainers, and pots you use should be dry. Avoid the temptation to wash things during the process! Keep paper towels handy and your efforts will be rewarded with a salve that is shelf-stable and potent.

• EXERCISE 9 •
Making Coconut Oil Salves

Beeswax salves are so easy, but using coconut oil is even easier! While I prefer olive oil for my beeswax salves (you can also use canola or almond), coconut oil has its benefits and makes a lovely ointment. A difference between the two is that beeswax salves will stay solid at higher temperatures than coconut will; it doesn't take much for coconut oil to liquefy, meaning that on a hot day, in a hot car, or on a shelf at a hot farmer's market, your coconut ointment will be pure liquid. It will resolidify when you refrigerate it, but it can be messy.

I like that coconut oil is light, but it's also slightly greasier than beeswax. Regardless, you can use any of the same herbs to make a coconut oil salve, and the process is a few steps shorter.

Suggested herbs to use with coconut oil include rose petals or cardamom. I once made a lovely coconut oil salve with rose petals and called it "Sanctuary Balm," as the scent was heavenly. Cardamom makes a bright, refreshing salve when infused with coconut oil and is a unique gift.

STEP 1: Scrape out all the solid coconut oil from a container into a saucepan. Gently heat it on the stovetop to liquefy; this will be quick.

STEP 2: Chop the herbs and add them to the container the coconut oil was in (unless it was plastic) or to any glass bowl, jar, or measuring cup where the oil and the herbs can sit for a few days undisturbed.

STEP 3: When the oil is liquefied, pull it from the heat and pour it into the container with the herbs. It will infuse directly in this container. Put the lid on, label it with the names of the herbs you used, and let it sit undisturbed for several days or a couple of weeks.

STEP 4: When you're ready, reheat the oil until it is liquid enough to pour through a strainer. Strain the herbs out, add a few drops of essential oil if you desire, and repackage your infused oil/coconut ointment into small salve jars. Label and store on a cool shelf or in the refrigerator.

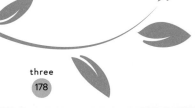

TIP 9

The Value of Small Batches

Think small—at least when you're making batches of herbal goodies. A little restraint goes a long way, especially when you're looking at a garden bursting with a bounty of herbs. Use pint jars instead of 2-quart jars and use small tins instead of 4-ounce glass containers. If you start small, you'll have more opportunity to experiment and will feel freer in your experimentation, letting the wild and reckless abandon of creativity run with you. Later, when you've perfected a recipe or nailed the process, you can confidently increase the size of your batches.

Lotions and Creams

Lotions and creams are a little different from salves. While salves (ointments) are made from herb-infused oil and beeswax or just coconut oil, lotions and creams incorporate water. They may be made with hydrosols (flower waters), plain water, or herb-infused water (tea), and they often include other watery ingredients such as aloe vera. Water in an oil-based salve would cause mold to grow, but in lotions and creams it makes the difference between an oily-feeling remedy and a creamy remedy that glides on the skin. Because of the water content, lotions and creams generally require refrigeration, and their shelf life is less than that of a salve—only a few months.

Herb-infused salves are healing for wounds and are called vulnerary. They cover a wound with a protective layer of wax, allowing the herbal chemicals to work against microorganisms, infection, and skin damage. Lotions and creams, however, are less vulnerary and more moisturizing, excellent for dry skin and dry hair.

 When you're healing a wound or an infection, use a salve; when healing dry skin, use a cream.

Lotions are basically creams that have more liquid added to them, and they are runnier. Creams can be very thick, while lotions are runny enough to be pumped through a lotion pump. Otherwise, they have the same ingredients.

When making a lotion or cream, use the same set of kitchen equipment for making salves and add a blender. Also, give yourself more time because the waxes require a period of cooling before the liquids can be added; you can place the blender in the refrigerator to speed this process or simply plan ahead, allowing for a waiting time in the middle of your project.

It's relatively simple to craft a lotion or cream. This is basically a blend of water and oil, and the ingredients are easy to substitute. Creativity reigns with lotions! Consider that you can make a passable lotion with nothing but oats and water (see exercise 14) and you'll sense how simple it can be. While they generally have the same ingredients, a lotion uses less beeswax and is allowed to remain liquid, while a cream tends toward being a more solid or pasty consistency.

• **EXERCISE 10** •

Making Lotion and Face Cream

Making a lotion or cream requires a blender. I've tried making lotions and creams with food processors and hand-held blenders, and they tend to frustrate the process. Be sure to have a long-handled rubber spatula ready, and it helps to have a working freezer available; make some room in it, if possible, because it may come in handy when you're wanting to speed along the process of cooling down hot ingredients by placing the blender in it.

This recipe is one I've used for years, adapted from fellow herbalists and edited with the input of my students every summer.

Waters

- $^2/_3$ cup hydrosol or herb-steeped tea
- $^1/_3$ cup aloe vera gel
- 5 to 10 drops essential oil (rose, lavender, lemon balm, or sustainably harvested frankincense)

Oils

- ¾ cup vegetable or nut oil (jojoba, sweet almond, or sunflower)
- $^1/_3$ cup coconut oil

- 3 to 4 tablespoons chopped beeswax (not beeswax beads)

STEP 1: In a saucepan on the stovetop, combine the oils first; melt the beeswax with the oils and then pour them directly into the blender. Now, allow them to cool; this will take time. Speed this process by placing the entire blender bowl into the freezer for twenty minutes or so.

STEP 2: Prepare the waters. Use straight hydrosol or brew a light tea with lavender or rose petals. Strain and set aside.

STEP 3: Once oils are cool, turn the blender on low speed and slowly add the waters. It will immediately turn creamy and the color will lighten. Blend until you achieve the consistency you want. Prepare a small amount of semi-soft melted beeswax to keep on hand if you find the lotion is too liquidy; this will solidify it more. Add more essential oils as the blender is running, if desired, but keep in mind that most face creams need to be mild and subtle, as a strong-smelling face cream can be harsh on the skin and eyes.

Spritzers

Another way to enjoy herbs is by making spritzers. These aren't the alcoholic drinks you find at summer parties—instead, they are fragrant little bottles of herbal waters that feel refreshing when sprayed or spritzed onto the body, especially on a hot day.

Spritzers are incredibly easy to make and are fun for kids to do—my kids have hosted a few spritzer-making afternoons where the kitchen becomes an aromatic laboratory littered with bottles, spray caps, labels, colored markers, and tiny bottles of essential oils. Each child goes home with one or two creations that last indefinitely and smell wonderful.

Because they don't need refrigeration, the spritzers can be used anywhere: keep them in your purse for on-the-go scent sprays, in the classroom to calm an upset child, or anywhere in the house for fragrance. One of my favorite places to keep them is in the fridge—not because they can go bad, but because when they are chilled they are wonderful to spray on the face and body on a hot day.

• EXERCISE 11 •
Making Spritzers

Spritzers only need two or three ingredients: water (distilled or not), essential oils, and—if desired—a little witch hazel. As we've mentioned, essential oils require a huge amount of plant material to yield a small amount of oil, so use them respectfully and be aware of how a company harvests the plants for their oils, choosing sustainable methods and reliable producers when possible. Witch hazel can be purchased at most pharmacies; be aware that retail witch hazel always contains 14 percent isopropyl alcohol, which is poisonous to consume, so be sure that anyone who may use the spritzer knows that it is for external use only.

STEP 1: Prepare your bottles by removing the spray caps and lining them up on the table. Consider which essential oils you will use: birch and balsam peru make a lovely forest-scented spritzer; catnip is quite exotic and refreshing; lemon and orange are upbeat; rosemary is traditionally used to help improve memory; lavender is soothing and calming; and rose is wonderful for grief and sadness, though pure rose essential oil is extremely expensive. I do not recommend using fragrance oils because these are often preserved or processed with petroleum and harmful chemicals that can be inhaled or absorbed through the skin. Try to purchase pure essential oils only, and use them respectfully.

STEP 2: In a four-cup glass or Pyrex measuring container, combine water (enough to fill your bottles, but no more) with four to five drops per cup of water of the essential oils. Whisk. To this add one to two teaspoons witch hazel and whisk some more. Smell the mixture and add more essential oil if necessary.

STEP 3: Pour the water and essential oil mixture into the bottles, whisking while pouring because the oils will naturally rise to the top of the water. Cap and label.

Instead of plain water, you may also use herbal tea, but be aware that the shelf life will be shortened; store in the refrigerator and check for mold after a few weeks.

Create an Herbal Bath Experience

Indulging in a hot bath can be incredibly healing, for both the body and the spirit. We often submerge our bodies into hot water to ease tension in our muscles and joints, and to let the heat melt away pain. We can also use the bathtub to inhale wonderful scents, to soften our skin, and to enjoy the aroma of fresh or dried plants. Create a healing bath experience with herbs using these ideas:

• EXERCISE 12 •
Making a Bath Tea

In a large two-handled pot on the stove, such as a large pasta pot or lobster pot, bring water to a boil. (The handles will help you safely carry the pot to the tub.) Add fresh or dried herbs, such as sprigs of thyme, stalks of catnip or peppermint, yarrow, fennel, rosemary, balsam fir, or eucalyptus. Consider rosemary, lavender, yarrow, sage, angelica, anise hyssop, lemon balm, catnip, plantain, and rose petals. Black birch leaves and twigs are anti-inflammatory, as are mustard seeds. Sliced ginger root is a great addition to reduce muscle tension.

Loosely cover the pot and brew these plants in the hot water as long as possible—from twenty minutes up to an hour. Meanwhile, run the bath and prepare the space.

I like to place a filled hot water bottle in the tub to act as a pillow so I have something to lean back on. Alternatively, soak a folded towel in the water as a pillow—but be sure you don't mind it changing color, as sometimes the herbs you use can stain fabrics. (They can also stain enamel, so do a test prior to filling the tub.) Place a large spaghetti strainer in the tub in preparation for pouring the tea through it.

Carefully carry the pot of tea to the tub and pour it through the strainer. Continue filling the tub with water and indulge in the bath while everything is still warm. Be sure to breathe in deeply and enjoy the full sensory experience of these fragrant and healing plants.

Alternatively, get two or three mesh tea balls and fill them with fresh or dried herbs, and toss them into the tub while the water is running. With each of these options, the fragrance is healing and the herbs are soothing to the skin.

Some tubs, especially porcelain, are susceptible to staining; be sure to clean the tub immediately after the bath to avoid damage or color stains from the herbal materials.

• EXERCISE 13 •
Making a Bath Garden

If you like the idea of bathing with plants, don't strain out the herbs—instead include them in the bathtub just as they are. You can bathe with sprigs of thyme, stalks of rosemary, and entire branches of catnip. Choose herbs that are fairly soft and swish them around while you're bathing in the hot water. Don't use rose stems since they have thorns, but rose petals are lovely and will stick to your body while you bathe. This is a lovely way to experience plants. Don't forget to use them to exfoliate your skin, too.

• EXERCISE 14 •
Making a Bath Lotion

Use raw oats to create a soothing lotion that is wonderful on the skin. Oats can be moistened and rubbed on the face at the sink for a quick revitalizing treat, or they can be added to the bath for a full-body soothing effect. Place a handful of oats in a muslin bag or simply in a strainer under the running tub faucet. In warm water, the oats will release a soupy, slippery "lotion" that is a good moisturizer for the skin. Afterwards, use the oats to scrub the tub; they can act as a sponge when you're done.

• EXERCISE 15 •

Enjoying a Foot Soak with Epsom Salt and Herbs

A foot soak is a great way to enjoy the healing properties of plants. Collect strongly fragrant herbs, such as mustard seed, eucalyptus, sliced ginger root, peppermint and spearmint leaves, catnip, rosemary, and sage. Crumble them (if dried) or coarsely chop them (if fresh) and place them in a large bowl or container to use as your foot tub. Add three to four tablespoons of Epsom salts to the herbs.

When you're ready, pull the foot tub up to your favorite chair, put on some good music or get your favorite book, wrap up with a blanket, and pour nearly hot water into the bowl. While the herbs are settling back down to the bottom—and infusing their properties into the water—relax. Test the temperature of the water, and when it's not too hot, gently lower your feet into it and sit back.

If you or a loved one can massage your calves while you're enjoying the foot bath, all the better. Because these herbs are good circulatory stimulants, this is a great time to breathe deeply and massage your muscles, releasing tension and stretching anything that might be tight.

Remedies for Internal Use

When we dive into the body—literally and metaphorically—things become much more complex. Our amazing bodies are made of tissues, organs, and systems that interact and relate in the most magnificent ways, usually unbeknownst to us and with great efficiency. Generally, there's not much for us to do but feed our bodies and exercise them regularly; everything else is done for us and proceeds quite normally ... that is, until something goes wrong. We become injured or stung by a bee or we eat too much sugar. We allow our stress level to skyrocket, which impacts the digestion or the skin or the heart, or something insidious and invisible interrupts our natural rhythms and we spend weeks or months in an effort to determine the cause, find a solution, and move forward.

Plants shine in these circumstances: they act as both nourishers and stabilizers when things are going well, and they are remedies when things go wrong. Plant medicines can help with both acute illnesses and chronic issues, and many people have found them to be more reliable and have fewer side effects than conventional or pharmaceutical drugs. Usually when we take herbs as medicine, we take them internally as a tea (infusion or decoction), a syrup, a tincture, a capsule, or a powder. We can also take herbal medicines internally as tinctures, vinegars, honeys, and milks—this versatility makes them incredibly useful for all ages and for people with dietary restrictions. Those who can't consume alcohol can take a vinegar tincture, and those avoiding sugars (found in honey, alcohol, or milk) can use powdered herbs as capsules, blended with water, or mixed into oatmeal.

Versatility, flavor, ease of use: all of these are benefits of herbal medicine that has made it a mainstay of traditional healing in cultures worldwide. Add to this the fact that herbal medicine is the people's medicine, and herbs grow locally and can be harvested easily, and we have a method of healing that is trustworthy, accessible, and encourages autonomy.

Using herbs internally requires a bit of forethought with regard to dosage and frequency. It's useful to know how much and how often, and while that is dependent largely on which herb you are taking, the following chart is a general guide to internal medicines for both adults and children.

DOSAGE AND FREQUENCY CHART
FOR INTERNAL REMEDIES

TYPE	ADULT	CHILD
	HOW MUCH HOW OFTEN	HOW MUCH HOW OFTEN
TEA (TONIC)	3–4 CUPS DAILY	1–2 CUPS DAILY
TEA (MEDICINAL)	2–3 CUPS DAILY	½–2 CUPS DAILY
TINCTURE (ALCOHOL)	¼ TEASPOON 3 TIMES DAILY	1/8 TEASPOON 3 TIMES DAILY
TINCTURE (VINEGAR)	1 TEASPOON 2–3 TIMES DAILY	½ TEASPOON 2–3 TIMES DAILY
INFUSED MILK	1 CUP 1 TIME, AT NIGHT	½ CUP 1 TIME, AT NIGHT
INFUSED HONEY	½–1 TEASPOON 2–3 TIMES DAILY	½–1 TEASPOON 2–3 TIMES DAILY
POWDER	1 TEASPOON 1–2 TIMES DAILY	½ TEASPOON 1–2 TIMES DAILY

The basic idea behind liquid internal remedies is that the herbal properties are infused (concentrated, extracted) into the liquid menstruum. When you brew a tea, you are infusing the water with the herbal properties; when you steep herbs into honey, vinegar, or alcohol, you are infusing that liquid with the herbal properties. When you strain the herbs out, you are getting rid of the fiber while the helpful chemicals (flavonoids, saponins, polyphenols, minerals, vitamins, alkaloids, tannins, etc.) stay in the liquid, which becomes your medicine.

So far, we've explored remedies for internal use that include water, and we will also feature some that use honey: infused honeys, syrups, and oxymels. But there are many more types of remedies that can be taken internally. In fact, there are a number of menstruua, or liquids, that can be the base of an infused herbal remedy. You can infuse water with herbs, and this becomes tea, of course, which is also called tisane, infusion, or decoction. You can infuse milk with herbs, and this becomes a delightful remedy: consider warm milk infused with chamomile for a sleepless child. You can also infuse herbs into vinegar, oil (for external use only, such as a massage oil), and grain alcohol. (See the liquid extracts chart on page 160.)

Alcohol Tinctures

Grain alcohol is an interesting beast. Do not confuse it with isopropyl alcohol, which is rubbing alcohol and cannot be consumed internally. Instead, grain alcohols are ethyl alcohol, which is the basis for most liquors such as vodka, whiskey, beer, and wine.

As a menstruum for herbal medicines (a liquid into which herbal chemicals can be extracted or infused), grain alcohol is very strong. In fact, water, milk, and honey are incredibly mild compared to grain alcohol, and they have a very short shelf life, whereas grain alcohol tinctures can last for years—even decades—unrefrigerated. Alcohol not only extracts the viable chemicals from the herbs, it also acts as an antibiotic of sorts, killing germs and keeping the remedy free from spoilage.

Because ethyl alcohol tinctures are so strongly concentrated and potent, only a tiny amount is needed as a medicinal dose. For example, a typical dose of herbal tea (tisane, infusion, or decoction) is three to four cups daily, while a typical dose of herbal alcohol tincture is only about twenty-five drops three times daily.

Almost any herb can be tinctured; I encourage you to start with the herbs on the easy list and experiment with them in very small batches. For instance, collect glass pint jars and, following the labeling guidelines discussed earlier, harvest four or five herbs at once and tincture them. You can combine them in the same jar, but if you're just starting out, I recommend keeping them separate. This allows you to observe their color and any changes, as well as determine how the herbs affect you when you take them for an illness.

making

Making an Herbal Tincture

I like the folk method of making tinctures: placing every-thing in a jar together and waiting for time to do its work. There are other methods: percolation, for instance, and also a method where you strain out the herbs, dry them, burn them, and add the ash to the tincture, which I've never tried, but it may be of interest to you if you want to experiment with salts and acids. For the folk method, you'll use minimal materials (herbs, glass canning jars, and alcohol); it's a basic philosophy that has served herbalists for centuries and produces a reliable, effective tincture.

STEP 1: **Choose Your Herbs.** As well, choose the parts of the herb you want to work with. Think about your end goal: do you need a remedy for a bronchial illness such as pneumonia? You might want to choose ginger, pleurisy root, elderberry, or thyme. Or if you want a remedy for a digestive illness such as ulcers, or digestive symptoms such as gas and bloating, you might choose chamomile, catnip, motherwort, or hops. Are you making a tincture to help you relax at night? Herbs for this tincture might include lavender, chamomile, hops, or holy basil. Your end goal will determine which herbs you use. (Check out the herbal properties chart on page 121; for additional instruction on how to determine an herb's actions and create an effective formula, see my book *An Herbalist's Guide to Formulary*.) Chop your fresh herbs coarsely or purchase dried herbs from a reputable source.

STEP 2: **Choose Your Menstruum, or Liquid.** You can infuse an herb into many different liquids; for instance, you can simmer lavender flowers in milk for a fragrant, soothing before-bed drink. In this case, milk is your menstruum. You can infuse dandelion roots in apple cider vinegar to use as an iron tonic; in this case, vinegar is your menstruum. When you're making a tincture, you'll use alcohols such as brandy, vodka, or whiskey. Alcohols create a potent remedy and also extend the shelf life, making a strong medicine that lasts a long time and is highly concentrated; you only need one-fourth teaspoon of herbal tincture for a dose, as opposed to several cups of herbal tea.

Consider different alcohols for different plant parts. Ethyl alcohols such as vodka and whiskey, for instance, are very strong and work great for tough roots, hard barks, dense seeds, and tough leaves. Conversely, they can be too much for the tender and ephemeral plant parts such as flower petals, which are happier with milder brandies and red or white wines. Purchase good-quality vodka for strong herbs or good-quality brandy or wine for milder herbs. Keep in mind that the shelf life for herbs tinctured in wine is not quite as long as that of stronger ethyl alcohol; whereas vodka tinctures can last up to a decade or even longer, wine tinctures, in my experience, seem to be potent only for two to three years.

Another liquid menstruum you may use is vegetable glycerin. This thick, highly sweet substance is composed of isolated vegetable fats, and it is a common ingredient in cosmetics and herbal preparations. It can be used topically, and it is often included in herbal tinctures because it acts as a solvent, much like alcohol. It can be mixed with alcohol in your tincture or you can use it alone, though I've found that homemade glycerin tinctures are less potent than alcohol tinctures. It has the consistency of syrup and can be added to tinctures for a sweet flavor and to improve the medicine's mouthfeel.

STEP 3: **Combine the Herbs and the Liquid.** If you're working with fresh plant material, fill a glass canning jar with your chopped plant materials. Fill it loosely and then press down and add more. Pour your selected liquid over the herbs and fill to within a quarter-inch of the top of the jar's rim. This will decrease the amount of oxygen in the jar and therefore decrease the likelihood of spoilage. Cap and shake the jar, then open it and add more liquid if needed. This provides a 1:1 ratio of herbs to liquid. If you're working with dried herbs, fill a glass canning jar only one-fifth of the way full; this provides a 1:5 ratio. Or fill it halfway full; this provides a 1:2 ratio. Because dried herbs have less water content than fresh, they are already more potent and you don't need as much to create a potent tincture.

STEP 4: **Wait.** Allow your tincture to sit, capped and labeled, on a pantry shelf where you can access it now and then to give it a shake. Watch for mold or for broken, dripping, or oozing jars.

Some herbalists like to make their tinctures by the lunar or solar cycles. To do this, harvest aerial (above-ground) plant parts on a full moon and tincture them immediately; let the tincture sit at least a month, going through the next full moon cycle. Sometimes one month is enough, but they can go six months or even a full year. To harvest underground plant parts (the roots), harvest on a new moon and follow the same cycle. Similarly, to harvest according to the sun, harvest on the summer solstice and decant at the winter solstice; this schedule accounts for the energy of the plants and the environment.

STEP 5: **Strain and Bottle.** You can use a tincture press if you like or you can use your hands to squeeze every drop out of the marc, or leftover herbal matter. You can also use a cheesecloth to keep small bits out of the finished tincture.

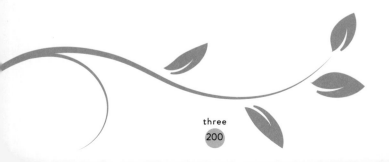

three

❀

Label That Jar!

Label your jars twice: once on the lid, using a permanent marker, and once on the side of the jar, using a piece of paper taped to the glass. Include specific information on each jar (of tincture, oil, etc.): the herb(s) inside, the date, the menstruum (liquid), and the batch number. It's also good to include the ratio of herbs to liquid (1:2 or 1:5, for instance), and if you fill more than one bottle with a particular blend, write "Bottle #1 of 3" so you'll know there are two more just like this one. This will keep your pantry organized, your remedies well-identified, and your final products safe, as you will know when they were made and how many were made at once. See page 147 for examples.

• EXERCISE 17 •

Making a Vinegar Tincture

Though the process is similar to making an alcohol tincture, the result is very different. While an alcohol tincture is incredibly concentrated and will last years, a vinegar tincture is less concentrated and more food-like and will last two to three years. As a strong acid, vinegar is very good at extracting minerals from substances (there is an old tradition of placing eggshells or animal bones into a jar of vinegar to extract the calcium). Vinegar can be relied upon to extract the calcium from raspberry leaf and the iron from nettle leaf or dandelion root.

Use vinegar tinctures when you want to avoid alcohol, when you'll be taking a remedy for a long period of time (several weeks or longer), and when you want to create other remedies or foods with it (such as honey-based oxymels and salad dressings).

STEP 1: **Select the Herbs.** Popular herbs to infuse into vinegar include garlic, motherwort, red clover, elderberry, fennel, nettle, and thyme. Fresh herbs are best; chop them and place them in a glass canning jar.

STEP 2: **Prepare the Vinegar.** While any vinegar will potentially work, apple cider vinegar is best. Avoid white vinegar and save the good balsamic for fruits and syrups. Apple cider vinegar provides enzymes, nutrients, and enough acid to make a successful tincture. In a small saucepan, gently heat the vinegar to warm it, but do not let it boil. Pour the vinegar over the herbs in the jar.

STEP 3: **Cap and Label.** Cap the jar with a plastic lid or a metal lid lined with wax paper, as vinegar will corrode a metal lid. Label, following the labeling guidelines previously listed, and store in a cool place such as a pantry shelf or cabinet. Because vinegar can ooze out of the jar, place a dish under the jar to catch any liquid and protect the shelf.

STEP 4: **Wait.** Allow the mixture to steep for four to six weeks. When it is ready, strain the liquid through a strainer and discard the herbs. Pour the liquid into labeled jars. Use glass dropper bottles if the vinegar will be a medicinal remedy; use salad dressing jars if you plan to add oils or spices to create a salad dressing (for every tablespoon of oil, add two to three tablespoons of infused vinegar).

Herbs and Honey

I love making infused honeys, which are honey remedies made by infusing (soaking, steeping, brewing, extracting) herbs into pure honey, creating a sweet, mild remedy that can be taken by the teaspoonful, stirred into tea, or spread onto toast. It can also be mixed with vinegar (infused or not), which is a sweet and tangy blend called an oxymel.

• EXERCISE 18 •

Making Infused Honey

STEP 1: **Choose Your Herbs.** Fragrant herbs are best: lemon balm, holy basil, lavender, spearmint, peppermint, and rose. Bitter or pungent herbs also work well in honey, as the honey makes them more palatable: motherwort, garlic, yarrow, and sage. Nettle works very well, too. I haven't tried sweet herbs such as licorice because it would seem the remedy would be too sweet, but feel free to experiment with whatever herbs you like. Chop the herbs coarsely and place them in a saucepan; make sure there is no extra water or moisture in the herbs, as water will spoil the honey. QUANTITY: you want to cover the bottom of the pan.

STEP 2: **Choose Your Honey.** Any pure, thin honey will do; avoid overly processed honey, honey with sugar water added, and thick honey such as buckwheat honey. Pour the honey over the herbs in the saucepan. QUANTITY: you want to cover the herbs completely plus about one inch of honey in the pan.

STEP 3: Place the saucepan on the countertop, cover with a lid, and let it sit overnight.

STEP 4: In the morning, place the saucepan on the stove and turn the heat on low. The goal is to liquefy the honey enough to pour it through a strainer. Do not simmer or boil the honey, just warm it.

STEP 5: Pour the honey and herbs through a strainer; use a cheesecloth or not. You may need to let the honey/herb mixture strain for an hour or more. Prop or hang the pot or strainer in a place where gravity can do its work for you. After an hour or so, squeeze as much honey as you can from the herbs, composting the herbs and preserving the honey.

STEP 6: Pour the now-infused, fragrant honey into a container such as a glass canning jar, and label it. Because there is no water added, this infused honey should be relatively shelf stable and will keep on the counter for several weeks. Alternatively, store the honey in the refrigerator for up to three months.

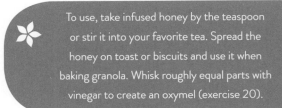

To use, take infused honey by the teaspoon or stir it into your favorite tea. Spread the honey on toast or biscuits and use it when baking granola. Whisk roughly equal parts with vinegar to create an oxymel (exercise 20).

Making Syrup

Another way to combine herbs and honey is to make syrup. A syrup combines a sweet substance, such as honey or sugar, with water or herbal tea. I've used maple syrup, too, but I prefer the honey and water combinations best. You can infuse the honey with herbs, or the water, or better yet, infuse both—this makes for a tasty and medicinal syrup that can be taken by the teaspoonful or stirred into tea or spread on toast or biscuits.

It's important to remember that because the honey is mixed with water, the shelf life is very short. Syrup must be refrigerated. (An infused honey with no water added is relatively shelf stable, as is an oxymel, but when you add water, you reduce the shelf life immediately.)

STEP 1: Gather your herbs. Choose fresh or dried, sweet or bitter, tangy or smooth. Any herb works in a syrup, though I tend to use bitter or pungent herbs in syrups because the sweet ingredients hide the bitterness. You can make rose syrup, lavender syrup, motherwort syrup, mint syrup, garlic syrup ... the choices are endless. If using fresh herbs, chop them coarsely and set aside about one cup. If using dried herbs, prepare about half a cup.

STEP 2: Gather your other materials: either one cup honey or sugar and one cup water. Be prepared to heat the mixture and whisk it.

STEP 3: Infuse the water or the honey (or both) with the herbs. If infusing the water, simply boil water and pour it over the herbs in a saucepan or teapot and brew as if you were brewing tea. If infusing the honey, start the night before for the best results, and follow the instructions in exercise 18.

STEP 4: Strain the water and/or the honey, then combine them in a saucepot. Over very low heat, gently whisk them together until you feel the consistency (and also the taste) are to your liking. If it's too thin, add more honey. If it's too thick, add more water. When you've reached the consistency you want, pour the syrup into bottles, label, and store in the refrigerator.

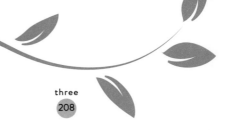

Making a Honey and Vinegar Oxymel

An oxymel is an exotic-tasting and incredibly easy remedy to create. It's one of my favorites because I love sweet and sour combinations, and that's exactly what an oxymel is. It can be a combination of lemon juice and sugar, for instance, or it could combine honey and apple cider vinegar. You could probably combine maple syrup with something sour, like lime juice, if you wanted. What's important is that you've infused some medicinal herbs into either the sweet or the sour. I usually infuse honey with herbs (such as garlic or motherwort) and infuse the vinegar with herbs (such as lemon balm, valerian, rose hips, etc.) for a doubly infused combination.

This is a remedy where you can let your creative genius run wild. You're in for a treat with this one because it is an unusually sensual remedy to make. By this I mean you can get enraptured with the tangy smell of the apple cider vinegar simmering on the stovetop, by the languid thickness of the honey as you stir it. Not to mention the stimulating scents of the herbs themselves—try using bright mint that will make your sinuses clear right open, bitter motherwort that sits on your tongue and causes you to salivate, or heady lavender that fills your brain with its own version of a thick fragrance. This is a remedy that invites us to experiment, to play with different herbs, and to make lots of various combinations. Above all, create something delicious that you will enjoy taking by the spoonful whenever you need it.

The method of taking an oxymel is quite easy: sip a spoonful of it. Alternatively, you can add it to a small bit of seltzer or soda, or to a small bit of elderflower liqueur for something similar to an herbal "shrub." It also makes a delicious salad dressing: simply pour it on your fresh salad along with a drizzle of olive oil or oil of your choice; it is especially tasty drizzled on fruit salads and even useful in any meat dish that requires a marinade.

STEP 1: Choose your herbs. An oxymel is a great place to use herbs that are generally too strong or bitter to use elsewhere, such as garlic, motherwort, yarrow, or wormwood. Because the sweet and sour taste is so prominent, you can hide those flavors that are usually considered unpleasant medicines. Oxymels are also a good remedy to take in the morning or during the day; because of the sugar, I don't usually take them at night. For this reason, here's a good place to use wake-up or energizing herbs such as eleuthero (Siberian ginseng) and schizandra. Finally, I think oxymels are a lovely place to use heart-healing herbs—those needed for both the circulatory system and good cardiovascular function, as well as those needed for emotional support of the heart. For instance, infuse hawthorn, rose petals, lemon balm, garlic, motherwort, prickly ash, and/or tulsi into your oxymel.

STEP 2: Decide whether you will infuse the sweet (honey, sugar, maple syrup) or the sour (vinegar, lemon juice) or both. If infusing honey, follow the instructions in exercise 18. Strain the herbs out and reserve the honey. If infusing the vinegar, chop your herbs and add them to a small saucepan. Pour in the vinegar and gently warm it on the stovetop. Do not allow it to boil, but let it heat for about fifteen minutes. Strain the herbs out and reserve the liquid.

STEP 3: In a glass bowl or large glass measuring cup, begin to combine them. I like to start small, so perhaps a half cup of honey mixed with a half cup

making

of vinegar. Taste this combination and see if you prefer it more sweet or more sour. Add accordingly, stirring and tasting as you go.

STEP 4: When you've achieved the flavor you like, bottle the oxymel in a glass jar or bottle, label it, and store it. Because there's no water, an oxymel can stay on the counter at room temperature, especially if you believe it will be used up within a week, but to guard against fermentation, I prefer to store it in the refrigerator. I've had oxymels ferment and explode, so refrigerating them seems wise. Use your oxymel within a few months.

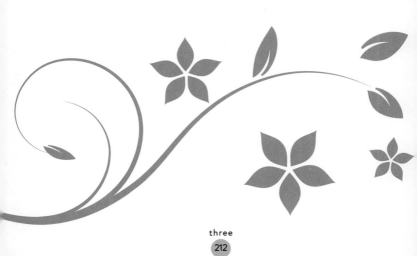

Making Fizzy Drinks

When you have an herbal syrup on hand, it's easy to add a little seltzer or carbonated water to it to make a soda-type drink. You can find flavored seltzers and pair them with your herbs: for instance, lemon seltzer with lemon balm syrup, lemon seltzer with hibiscus syrup, or blood orange seltzer with ginger-motherwort syrup. It's also easy to add liqueur or cordial to these sodas; my favorite is elderberry flower liqueur, which pairs amazingly with almost anything. Also, infused vinegars pair well with blackberry, strawberry, or fig syrups and with mint, rose, lemon balm, lemon verbena, or elderberry syrups. It's hard to go wrong; just blend the drinks until you reach the sparkling sweet balance you want.

To begin, start with one cup of seltzer and slowly add one-fourth cup of syrup to it, tasting as you go. You may go up to equal amounts depending on how sweet you want it. If you're adding liqueur or vinegar to the beverage, add these one tablespoon at a time, to taste.

TIP II

Host a "Making" Party

Decide what you'll make and have all the ingredients ready. Invite friends and offer easy finger foods that can be eaten around the various tables you'll have set up. Provide cups for hot or iced tea and plenty of pitchers or carafes for self-serving. Be sure enough products are made so that everyone goes home with several of their own. Provide ribbons, labels, string or twine, jars, bottles, stickers, and decorations along with ingredients. For instance, prepare one work table with salve-making equipment (including a hot plate and extension cord), jars, lids, and a cutting board for beeswax. On another table, a large, deep bowl for mixing dried teas, with tins or bags and labels. Making parties are also great opportunities to make syrups, grind herb salts, and bottle massage oils.

FOUR

USING AND SHARING

Congratulations! You've proceeded from growing and harvesting to making, and now you have wonderful herbal remedies that you can use. This is a fun part of herbal crafting—actually putting your creations to use and finding function and value in them.

There are as many ways to use herbs and herbal remedies as there are herbalists, and that creativity is part of the appeal. Just because someone else uses their yarrow salve on wounds doesn't mean you have to; you can use it as a boot polish, if you would like—in fact, though this isn't medicinal, it's really effective, and I have many pairs of leather boots that enjoy their yearly wipe-down with an oil and beeswax herbal ointment. It keeps the leather supple and inhibits the growth of mold or mildew on boots that have been sitting in a closet for months.

The key to enjoying herbal remedies on a regular basis is to keep them handy. Rather than storing remedies in a cabinet or drawer, keep them on an open shelf, in your purse, on your desk, etc. Keep them somewhere easy to reach for; you'll use them frequently. This will accomplish several things: the remedy gets used and not wasted, you feel satisfied using something you made, and you learn how the remedy acts in or on your body so you can make adjustments the next time you craft this remedy to make it even more functional and relevant.

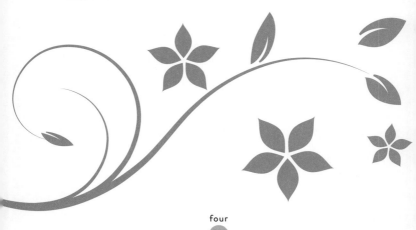

TIP 12

Keeping Herbs
Fresh in the Kitchen

After harvesting parsley, dill, fennel, cilantro, or lemon balm for use in culinary or medicinal applications, keep them fresh by placing the stalks in a glass of water and snipping off the leaves as you need them. Stored this way, fresh herbs will keep about five days. Alternatively, dampen a paper towel, gently wrap the stalks of herbs in the towel, and place it in an open plastic bag. Store this in the refrigerator and use within three days.

Using Fresh Herbs in the Kitchen

In the growing months, fresh herbs are available for the picking. Try these ideas to get the most out of your fresh herbs:

- Harvest your herbs by the whole stem and keep them in a glass jar or vase right on the counter or on the windowsill above the sink. Train yourself to snip off leaves for cooking; snip cilantro, lavender, parsley, sage, catnip, and lemon balm.

- Snack on them; I love snacking on fennel fronds or seeds.

- Grow the herbs in small pots in the kitchen: nettle, catnip, mint, chamomile, and yarrow all grow well in small pots and can be used conveniently.

- Think of using fresh herbs in every meal of the day. Get in the habit of snipping vitamin C–rich parsley into your eggs in the morning, into your hummus at lunch, and onto your meat and fish at dinner. Dill, fennel, mint, rosemary, thyme, and sage all contribute flavor and minerals to meals and

are especially good fresh. All parts of fennel
can be used: the fronds, flowers, seeds, and
bulb. Keep it handy so you can throw it in
everything, especially sausage and meat
dishes.

And then, of course, cooking with freshly harvested
herbs from the garden or the wild is fun. If you're new
to this, try using rose petals, as they are fairly easy to
come by in the growing season. Just make sure they haven't
been sprayed with any chemicals. Harvest the petals
and use them in ice cubes (see exercise 22), rice pudding,
shredded into your oatmeal, baked with your granola,
and used as a garnish on almost anything, especially salads.
Also try these methods with violet flowers and calendula
flowers.

Creative Ways to Use Brewed Tea

In chapter 3 you learned to brew tea. There are so many
ways to use tea in addition to drinking it. You can drink
it, of course, and enjoy it for its flavor and its medicinal
value, but there are other ways to use herbal tea:

- Pour herbal tea infusions onto potted
  houseplants.

- Pour herbal tea infusions onto garden plants.

- Ferment a large batch of tea in a bucket to use as fertilizer in the garden.

- Bathe your dog or cat with herbal infusion (good herbs for "shampoo tea" include calendula, spearmint, lemon balm, and rose); keep it out of the eyes, and rinse thoroughly.

- Use brewed tea in place of water in lotions (see exercise 10).

- Use brewed tea in place of water in syrups (see exercise 19).

- Use brewed tea to dye fabrics and in artistic projects such as painting and dying Easter eggs. Experiment with calendula for light yellow, yellow dock root for amber, elderberry for pink, hibiscus flower for pink, and nettle leaf for green.

Another way to use leftover brewed tea is to make ice cubes.

• EXERCISE 22 •
Making Ice Cubes

To those colorful teas you can add colorful ice cubes! If you have a freezer, these are very easy to make. Simply collect fresh flowers such as violets, calendula, roses, daisies, black cumin, elder, or lavender, or collect small leaves such as spearmint. Fill an ice cube tray half full with water or herbal tea, tuck a flower or leaf into each slot, then carefully fill with more water. You may need to poke the flowers in a bit to make them stay submerged.

Place the tray in the freezer and check on it after about fifteen minutes; resubmerge the flowers if necessary, then return the tray to the freezer until the cubes are completely frozen. When you're ready to serve tea, select a clear glass pitcher or decanter and add your ice cubes to the tea. Add additional slices of lemon, limes, and oranges and even full fennel fronds if you're feeling adventurous.

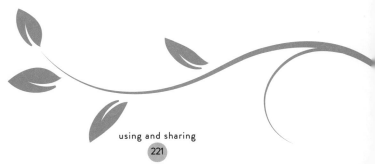

Sharing Your Creations
Make Gift Baskets

Herbal remedies are essential for those who are sick, injured, or wanting to keep themselves healthy. A well-stocked pantry or medicine cabinet is a gift in itself! Herbal remedies make wonderful gifts in so many ways, allowing us to be creative and have fun while the beneficiaries get something useful, beautiful, and healing.

Someone will greatly appreciate the lip balm you make them or the little bottle of infused vinegar or the lavender sachet. Herbs lend themselves to everything from candles to cabinets and from incense to intention cards. Here are some ideas for gifting whole baskets of goodies to those you love throughout the year.

• EXERCISE 23 •
The Summer Basket

Summer baskets make wonderful gifts for lots of reasons; you hardly need an excuse to give one, but here are several: summer guests and visitors at your house, baskets in an inn or hotel for vacationers, first aid baskets for your camper, a scented basket of goodies for your dog, etc.

STEP 1: **Determine the Giftee.** Will it be your neighbor, your teenager going off to camp, or a guest coming to visit?

STEP 2: **Collect and/or Make Items.** Collect and/or make items that will fill a small basket full of goodies for the summer. Think outside the bottle and include things that smell good, feel good on the skin, and even taste good. To make it well-rounded, also include non-herbal items or things you didn't make, such as a bandana, store-bought sunscreen, wet wipes, soap, and a good book. Handmade ideas include:

- FIRST AID OINTMENT: Made with anti-inflammatory and antimicrobial cultivated herbs such as rosemary, sage, eucalyptus, ginger, yarrow, arnica, and plantain. Follow the instructions in exercise 8 for beeswax salves.

- SCENTED SPRITZER: Made with water, a little witch hazel, and essential oils of your choice for scent; good ones include lemon or lavender.

- HAND LOTION: These have a short shelf life, so include a note to keep it refrigerated. Follow the instructions in exercise 10.

- OXYMEL: Though oxymels are wonderfully medicinal and could be included in the basket to ward off illness and keep your loved one healthy, it can also be used as a tangy and delicious salad dressing. Follow the instructions in exercise 20.

STEP 3: **Wrap It Up.** Find an airy basket at a thrift store and line it with a light and breezy scarf or a light tablecloth that could inspire a picnic. Place the larger items first and fill in the holes with the smaller items; better yet, wrap the smaller items in a bit of paper so they don't get lost or overlooked.

• EXERCISE 24 •
The Camp Basket

If your giftee's summer includes camping, this basket of herbal remedies will keep them healthy and happy:

STEP 1: Collect and/or make items that will fit in a small day pack or fanny pack, which will be your basket. Include extra (non-herbal) items such as a bandana, a washcloth, and paper and pen.

STEP 2: Include remedies that are useful and natural; being in the woods means a camper doesn't want detergents, fake scents, or other harmful chemicals that could spoil pristine waters or contaminate the air. Ideas include:

- INSECT REPELLENT: Bug repellent need not contain harmful DEET. Instead, fill a spray bottle with pure water, a little witch hazel, and essential oils traditionally used to keep insects at bay, including lemongrass, lemon verbena, mint, oregano, basil, camphor, eucalyptus, and citronella. Instead of water, you could begin your insect repellent with an infusion of herbs such as rosemary and tansy, then add the witch hazel and essential oils. Either way, your camper will smell great (to humans) and repellent (to insects). Label the bottle carefully.

- FIRST AID OINTMENT: When making ointments for the camper (following the instructions in exercise 8), pour the oil-beeswax mixture into a tin instead of a glass container. Use herbs such as yarrow, rosemary, sage, and elder leaf to make your first aid remedy extra potent; these herbs offer antimicrobial properties as well as analgesic, anti-inflammatory, and astringent actions, helpful when a camper suffers an injury or gets a rash.

- LIP BALM: When making this (following the instructions in exercise 8), pour the oil-beeswax mixture into a tube or tin.

- IMMUNE SUPPORT TINCTURE: Made with herbs such as echinacea, garlic, rose hips, and sage. Follow the instructions in exercise 16.

• EXERCISE 25 •
The Off-to-College Basket

When kids go away to school, they will quickly see the value of keeping healthy and will appreciate many of the herbal supports listed in this book. They'll also want things they can easily keep in their dorm room or back-pack. If they have access to a hot water kettle, a tea will

four

make a great addition to this basket; you may also want to include a small thermos in the gift.

Ideas for the college student's basket:

- FIRST AID OINTMENT: Especially useful will be an ointment made with herbs that soothe burns, such as plantain and mallow, or herbs that induce sleep, such as lavender, that can be gently rubbed onto the student's temples or wrists at bedtime. Follow the instructions in exercise 8.

- IMMUNE SUPPORT TINCTURE (made with herbs such as echinacea, garlic, rose hips, and sage). Follow the instructions in exercise 16.

- TEA. Consider the following blends for your students, and include a small thermos and/or a tea strainer:

  A SOOTHING NIGHT-TIME TEA: Include herbs such as chamomile, lemon balm, catnip, lavender, and holy basil.

  AN ENERGIZING MORNING TEA: Include herbs such as spearmint, peppermint, ginger, nettle, eleuthero (Siberian ginseng), and green tea.

A NOURISHING MINERAL-RICH TEA: Include
nettle, alfalfa, lemon balm, oatstraw, rose
hips, and fennel.

A STRESS-REDUCING TEA FOR ANXIETY
AND TEST-TAKING: Include lemon balm,
motherwort, passionflower, holy basil,
lemon verbena, rose petals, and eleuthero
(Siberian ginseng).

- OXYMEL: Bottled in a small one- or two-
ounce bottle with a dropper, an oxymel can
easily fit into a backpack and be a portable
source of tangy medicine. Make it with
motherwort for anxiety, or with rose hips
for extra vitamin C throughout the day.

- SPRITZER: Dorms can be smelly places; send
your student the gift of fragrance. Spritzers
contain germ-fighting essential oils, so
they can be sprayed on the body as well as
on surfaces such as doorknobs to increase
sanitation.

- LIP BALM, which can be in a typical lip balm
tube or a small salve tin.

• EXERCISE 26 •

The Mother's Day Basket

Indulge your mom or mother-in-law with lovely herbal gifts that come from the heart. There are a few themes she might like:

The "I Love You with My Whole Heart" Basket

This basket could include:

- heart-healing and strengthening herbs and foods, such as a motherwort tincture or oxymel
- an oatstraw blend infusion
- a rose spritzer

The "Indulge Yourself" Basket

- a scented lotion or face cream; consider lovely scents such as lemon balm, roses, lavender, or even cardamom
- a scented spritzer; add a note to her bottle that encourages her to keep it in the fridge so that it's cool when she uses it on a hot day
- lip balm

A Floral Basket

- rose or lavender lotion or face cream (follow the instructions in exercise 10)
- rose or lavender tea blend (include a small thermos, tea cup, or strainer)
- rose or lavender tea towels
- rose or lavender sachet to be tossed into a drawer or closet or into her purse
- rose or lavender potpourri
- rose or lavender soap
- rose or lavender spritzer (follow the instructions in exercise 11)

• EXERCISE 27 •
The Get-Well Basket

If you're gifting someone who has been ill, has spent some time in the hospital, has had an injury, or is recovering from an illness or from being the caretaker of someone in need, this basket can be both medicinal and comforting.

It can be nice to include an eye or neck pillow—sometimes these are scented and filled with buckwheat or rice so they can be heated in the microwave to soothe tense facial muscles and induce relaxation. It can also be thoughtful to include wet wipes, tea cup, mug, thermos, and a thick washcloth.

Those who spend a lot of time in hospitals wash their hands frequently and have dry hands; a gift of herbal lotion with a pair of soft gloves is appreciated. Include a good book with a bookmark and a few candles for when they are recovering at home.

The get-well basket can include:

- TEA. Consider soothing herbs such as chamomile, fennel, ginger, catnip, lavender, holy basil, etc. Make the blend and label it, and include a tea strainer.

- POWDERS: Because high-quality powders are difficult to make from home-grown plants (due to both quantity and quality), and because they're easy to find at most grocery stores and markets, purchase a few powders to keep in your kitchen. Good ones to have on hand are ginger, cinnamon, and turmeric; these are easy to find and fairly inexpensive.

    If you've grown your own plants, especially easy-to-dry herbs such as roses and lemon balm, try drying them and running them through a spice grinder. Sift the powder to remove chunks, and store the powder in tiny glass jars.

Tuck a small jar of herbal powder into a gift basket with instructions on how to use it. For instance, a spoonful of turmeric, cinnamon, and allspice powders can be sprinkled into a bowl of oatmeal or a pot of spaghetti sauce. A spoonful of elderberry powder can be stirred into a jar of apple cider or orange juice in the morning for immune support. A spoonful of cinnamon, ginger, and allspice can be a ready-made blend for making apple pie, cookies, or other feel-good treats.

When purchasing powders, shop at a store you trust for high-quality products; low-quality lookalikes and substitutes are sometimes sold as the real thing because so many medicinal plants are overharvested or rare. Purchase both powders and dried herbs from sources that guarantee organically grown and fair-trade equivalent growing and harvesting conditions; this helps guard against contaminants. Also, try to support local farms as much as possible.

- SPRITZERS: For those recovering from an illness—and still on pharmaceutical medications that may have the risk of contraindications—the sense of smell is often one of the few safe things in which they can indulge. Your giftee can spritz themselves and their bed with a lovely spritzer made with lavender, roses, lemon verbena, patchouli, sustainably harvested sandalwood, or balsam fir. Follow the instructions in exercise 11.

- HERBAL MASSAGE OIL: Use a base of carrier oils such as jojoba, kukui, sweet almond, or sunflower oil. In a glass bowl with tall sides (a large Pyrex measuring cup works well), whisk the carrier oils with a few drops of essential (concentrated) oils such as sustainably harvested sandalwood, palo santo, cinnamon, vanilla, birch, balsam peru, and balsam fir for a lovely scented massage oil. Your giftee can receive a massage or use the oil on their feet or legs—ideal for someone who has been caring for another person by lifting or walking.

- FIRST AID SALVE: Those who have had surgery will appreciate a good herbal first aid ointment, which can be applied to those areas healing from surgical wounds. First aid ointments are extremely helpful for women who have had chemotherapy or radiation for breast cancer as it strengthens the skin and repairs damaged tissues. Include healing herbs such as calendula, yarrow, plantain, mallow, elder leaf and flower, and rose petal. Follow the instructions in exercise 8.

- BATH INDULGENCES: Once the bandages come off and one can bathe, indulging in a soothing bath can calm the nerves and lift the spirits. Include in the basket several things that can go in the bathtub:

A LARGE STRAINER (MESH BALL) for straining tea that can hold herbs in the bath water; the bathtub, in essence, becomes a big teacup in which your giftee can soak his or her body.

SPRIGS OF FRESH OR DRIED HERBS such as thyme, fennel, tansy, rosemary, and sage; these can be swished in the water to release their scent.

CANDLES to go on the sides of the tub.

A WASHCLOTH AND A SPRITZER can round out this lovely basket.

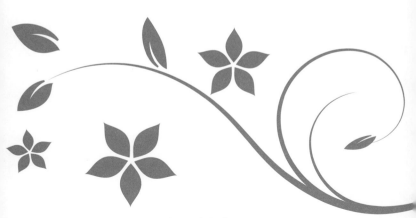

TIP 13

Keeping Spritzers in the Fridge

If you are gifting a fragrant spritzer—whether lavender, rose, catnip, eucalyptus, lemongrass, or other scent—tell your giftee to keep it in the refrigerator to use on hot days. A light spray on the face and neck with a cool spritzer feels wonderful in the summer months.

Using Essential Oils

The idea of gift baskets brings us to the use of essential oils. An essential oil (also called a volatile oil) is made of certain chemicals in the plant, terpenes, that provide the smell. When we inhale a stem of rosemary, we are smelling the essential oils. These oils are so light they evaporate easily, rising with the water in a distillation machine to create a pure product that can be captured and bottled. When collected with the water, it is called a hydrosol, or flower water. When the oils are skimmed off the top and collected separately, it is called the essential oil.

This oil is very potent. If you've ever used or watched a demonstration of a distillation machine (a "still"), you'll know that it can take handfuls, pounds, or even tons of plant material to yield only a very little essential oil. When using a home distiller, you can harvest basketfuls of plants and yield only a few drops of essential oil; when commercial distillers do this, they harvest literal tons of plants to yield only a few quarts of essential oil, which are bottled in tiny bottles and sold by the dram, by the half ounce, or by the ounce. This material is precious; we do not want to overharvest our plants in the process of creating essential oils. Unfortunately, this is exactly what is happening to some of the most fragrant and precious plants on earth, such as sandalwood and frankincense. The demand for these incredible fragrances is so high that we are at risk of harvesting these plants to extinction. For this reason alone, it is worthwhile to exercise restraint and educate ourselves about the essential oil manufacturing process.

It's also important to recognize that essential oils are potent in and on our bodies and must be used with caution and, again, restraint. Essential oils are incredibly antibacterial and antifungal, making them useful in salves and remedies that fight infection. Some people even consume them internally, but I've never recommended this as I believe essential oils are toxic internally and damage the liver, which is tasked with removing wastes from the blood. Instead, use essential oils topically and include them in spritzers, salves/ointments, and soaps, but they should never be included in tinctures, teas, oxymels, or any other remedy that you ingest.

For these reasons, I'm not recommending that you include bottles of essential oils in your gift baskets. While it may be compelling to toss in a lovely smelling fragrant essential oil such as lavender for your giftee, I think working with herbs comes with a responsibility toward safety and education, and handing someone a bottle of essential oil who has not been educated about its use, history, and function can lead to trouble. Instead, gift your student, mother, or friend with remedies you've crafted (using essential oils or not), and save the essential oils for use in projects where you can be discerning and careful.

Finally, wrap all these gift baskets with love and give them freely; sharing herbal remedies and goodies spreads not only good cheer but also the idea of connection with plants, which can be eye-opening for someone and can be the beginning of a life-long love affair.

Using Fresh Herbs as Medicines

Using herbs need not be restricted to dried herbs, capsules, or pills you purchase from the store. If you've gotten this far in this book, you've gardened, grown, and harvested, and now you're using those wonderful herbs and remedies for health and well-being. Fresh herbs can be placed in a glass of water on the windowsill and snipped from for cooking; fresh herbs can be mashed with a spoon or in a mortar and pestle and applied to the face or the skin—rose petals and cucumber-scented borage flowers make a lovely "mask" for the face. Fresh herbs can hang in lovely bunches from the rafters to dry

(I generally use these for looks; if you want to appropriately dry your herbs for medicinal use, see exercise 4.)

One more way to use fresh herbs—and to enjoy those ephemeral gifts of plants while they're fresh and succulent—is to make poultices with them. A poultice is an application of fresh plants on the skin. It's a great remedy for a wound, for instance, or for sore muscles. Poultices are a common remedy when camping because all they require is a freshly harvested leaf (or pine needles, a comfrey leaf, yarrow, or plantain weeds) and water.

A number of topical applications can be made similar to poultices, and all are worth experimenting with, even if you don't have a wound, simply so you can know the process and be ready when it is needed. The best of these are a spit poultice, a compress, and a regular poultice.

• EXERCISE 28 •
Making and Using a Spit Poultice

Saliva is a great liquid for healing wounds, and chewing a leaf and then placing it on a wound has got to be the oldest form of healing. Some herbs are soothing to wounds, others will fight infection, and some are actually drawing agents that pull things from the body. Plantain is a drawing herb, and I've used it countless times to draw bee venom out from a honeybee sting. Simply harvest ten to twenty plantain leaves and chew them one at a time. When the leaf starts softening in your mouth (after only a few seconds of chewing), take it out and place it on the sting. Immediately you will feel the leaf grow hot; not only is it absorbing the heat from your wound, but it's also drawing out the venom. Discard the spent leaf and chew another, then apply it. After going through the ten to twenty leaves, the sting should no longer hurt or itch. You can also apply this method to simple cuts using plantain, yarrow, or mint.

• EXERCISE 29 •

Making and Using a Compress

This requires a heating source and a pan to which you can add water. If you're camping, simply build up the fire. If you have access to a kitchen, choose a small to medium saute pan with low sides. You'll also need scraps of fabric, such as strips of cotton or flannel, to act as a bandage.

Pour one to two cups of water into the pan and heat on medium heat. Meanwhile, chop the herbs you want to use. If making a compress for an abrasion, for instance, you can select mallow leaf, plantain, yarrow, sage, calendula flowers, mullein, comfrey, pine, balsam fir, hemlock tree, bee balm flowers, elderflowers, elder leaf, etc. Avoid highly fragrant plants such as lemon grass, mint, or citrus peel because these can sting the fresh wound.

Add the herbs (whole, chopped, or shredded) to the pan of water and heat for ten to twenty minutes. You're basically making a tea, but this will be for topical use.

Dip the cloth into the water and soak up as much "tea" as you can. Wring gently and place on the abrasion. Though it's messy, this should feel warm and soothing. Reapply the cloth to the hot water when it cools, and keep the wet cloth on the abrasion as long as possible, ten to fifteen minutes. Repeat several times a day.

The advantages to a compress are that you're not placing the herbs directly on the abrasion—only the wet cloth. This is a benefit when you're working with children who may be squeamish about the idea of plants on their bodies or when you're working with plants that have hairs or bits that could lodge in the abrasion itself. Additionally, compresses are easy to clean up.

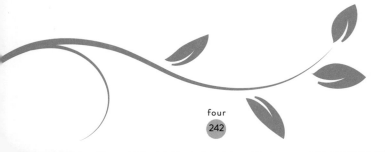

• EXERCISE 30 •
Making and Using a Regular Poultice

To take the concept of the compress one step further, make a regular poultice. Follow the steps for making a compress, choosing from the list of herbs in exercise 29 and heating them in the water. Instead of dipping a cloth in the water, however, pull the herbs themselves from the pan and place them directly on the wound. This can be repeated as long as the water stays hot, but the real advantage is in wrapping the plants on the skin to keep them there long-term. Layer the plant material thickly onto the wound and use plastic wrap or tape a cloth around the area to keep the plants in place. This can be left on for several hours, and the remedy may be repeated two to three times per day.

The advantage of a poultice is that the person carries the remedy with them—it's wrapped so you don't need to sit still. Also, the wet, warm plant gets to do its job over a period of time, leading to a more saturated effect and a deeper healing. The only downside is that certain plants (such as mullein or comfrey) have minute hairs that can lodge in a wound; consider this when choosing between a compress or a poultice. Also, avoid comfrey leaf on punctures because this herb has the amazing ability to heal the surface extremely quickly, leaving open areas beneath the surface vulnerable to infection.

Storing Your Remedies

Let's go through the list of remedies and goodies you've made throughout this book and detail the best way to store them.

Freshly Harvested Nettle Leaves

Dry them (as described in chapter 2) and store in a paper bag wrapped inside a plastic bag. Shelf life is one year for whole leaves, two to three months for crumbled or chopped leaves.

Freshly Harvested Roots

Dry them thoroughly (as described in chapter 2) and store in a paper bag wrapped inside a plastic bag or in a glass jar with a tightly fitted lid. Shelf life is one year for whole roots, two to three months for chopped roots.

Hot Tea, Sun Tea, and Iced Tea

Store your freshly brewed hot tea in a thermos for up to twenty-four hours; store your iced tea in the refrigerator for up to twenty-four hours.

Beeswax Salves

Store these at room temperature (do not keep them in a hot car)—a pantry shelf or cabinet is a good place. Shelf life for most beeswax salves is one to two years. You'll know it's gone bad when it loses its pleasant smell and the texture is rubbery instead of creamy.

Coconut Oil Salves

Store these at room temperature in cool climates or in the refrigerator in warm climates. The natural tendency of coconut oil is to be liquid. To maintain it as a salve, keep it cool or chilled. Shelf life is six to twelve months.

Lotion and Face Cream

Because these have water in them, they have a fairly short shelf life of three to six months. Store them on a counter or shelf away from direct sunlight, preferably in the refrigerator.

Spritzers

Though these are mostly water, I like to preserve them with witch hazel, which extends their shelf life. Stored on a pantry shelf, they will last several years. Stored in the refrigerator, they will last even longer.

Infused Honey

Honey generally has a long shelf life, and even when it's infused with herbs it is fairly stable, lasting six to twelve months in a container with a tightly fitted lid. However, adding water to it to make a syrup (or leaving the lid off in a humid room) will greatly reduce the shelf life to only a few days. Honey is humectant, soaking up water, so be sure to keep it properly lidded.

Honey and Vinegar Oxymel

Apple cider vinegar (and most other vinegars) are highly acidic and shelf-stable. An oxymel made with honey and vinegar will last six to twelve months when kept at room temperature on a pantry shelf or counter.

Ice Cubes

If you make herbal ice cubes and don't plan to use them immediately, store the whole ice cube tray (or crack the cubes out of it) in a plastic bag that seals, and keep it in the freezer for up to three months.

Syrups

Because of the water content, syrups fade quickly. Store them in the refrigerator and use them within three days.

Fizzy Drinks

Consume within twenty-four hours.

Foot Soak with Epsom Salts

Enjoy this immediately; do not store it for later use.

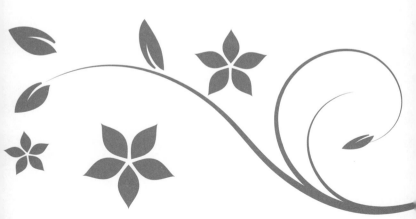

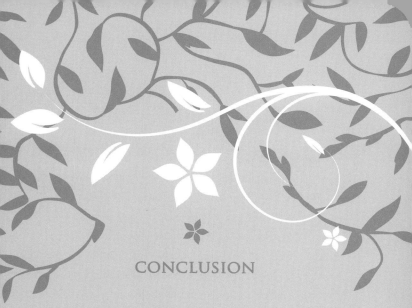

CONCLUSION

I used to find myself, in the cold days of January and February, cuddled up in bed with lots of fluffy blankets and maybe a cat or a dog or a child or two, reading seed catalogs and dreaming of next summer's garden. I'd turn the pages from herbs to flowers to potatoes to vegetables, circling gorgeous illustrations and admiring descriptions that brightened my imagination. In March or April a small box of seed packets would arrive. I loved the feel of the paper, the sound of seeds rustling inside. I'd fill the seed trays on the porch, and water and tend and spread straw around veggies and herbs; my family was rewarded with good things to eat and herbs for salves.

As you move forward, give yourself the time and space to appreciate the plants. Flowers work their magic regardless of whether they're infused in oil in our kitchens or simply looked at or smelled while they're growing. Their presence is healing.

The hands-on experience of harvesting and crafting with plants is fun. Recently I joined a group of friends for a "making" party; we assembled jars with lids and labels, brought crocks of long-handled spoons to the table, and stacked our bottles of vegetable and seed oils ready for use. We also took time to sit with each other, our feet in bowls of hot water, relaxing and sharing stories and asking each other about life's aspirations. Herbalism is the art and science of plants, but healing is so much more. There are as many ways to enjoy and use herbs as there are herbs for health and happiness!

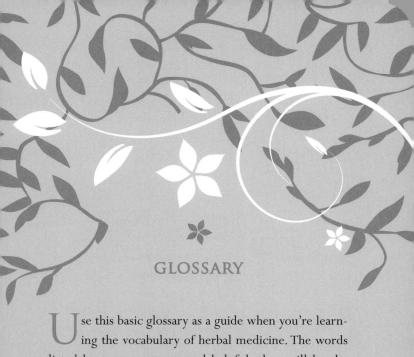

GLOSSARY

Use this basic glossary as a guide when you're learning the vocabulary of herbal medicine. The words listed here are common and helpful; they will be the basis of your understanding of the effects, properties, or actions of medicinal plants.

ANALGESIC: eases or relieves pain. Lavender and valerian can be analgesic.

ANTIMICROBIAL: a catch-all term that refers to a plant's ability to fight or kill pathogens. Can relate to antibacterial, antifungal, antiparasitic, antiviral, etc. Garlic and yarrow are strong antimicrobial herbs.

AROMATIC: a plant that is highly fragrant (i.e., its flowers or leaves smell strongly) is generally a good plant for the nervous system, the respiratory system, and the digestive system. Aromatics include spearmint, catnip, lemon balm, anise hyssop, and lavender.

ASTRINGENT: drying. Astringent plants will dry excess moisture and are effective on weepy skin conditions such as poison ivy. Lavender, rosemary, yarrow, and sage are astringent.

BITTER: possessing a bitter flavor when eaten. Bitter herbs often support digestive health and are used to ease gas and indigestion. Turmeric, chamomile, motherwort, calendula, and dandelion are bitter.

CARMINATIVE: soothing to the stomach. These herbs are often aromatic or bitter, and they ease gas, bloating, indigestion, diarrhea, and constipation. Lemon balm, catnip, ginger, holy basil, and fennel are carminative.

COUGH SUPPRESSANT: an herb that soothes spastic coughing and eases lower respiratory spasms. Elderberry, elecampane, thyme, and mallow are cough suppressant.

DECOCTION: similar to an infusion, a decoction is a process of brewing herbs in water to extract their properties. In a decoction, you brew the harder and denser parts of a plant, such as the roots, bark, and seeds; a lidded pot of water is brought to a simmer and kept simmering for twenty to thirty minutes or left to sit overnight on the counter. It is then strained and drunk as a strong tea. Avoid using bitter herbs in this process.

DEMULCENT: soothing and cooling; used internally. Often used to soothe heartburn, ulcers, or inflammation. Rose, lemon balm, self-heal, and plantain are demulcent.

ELECTUARY: powdered herbs blended into honey. Can be eaten by the spoonful, spread onto toast, or stirred into tea.

EMOLLIENT: soothing and cooling; used externally. Often used to ease rashes, eczema, psoriasis, and burns. Rose, lemon balm, lavender, jewelweed, St. John's wort, violet, black cumin, and borage are emollient.

EXPECTORANT: causes the lungs to contract or cough, releasing phlegm. Helpful during wet coughs. Elderberry, thyme, anise hyssop, angelica, and pleurisy root are expectorant.

GALACTAGOGUE: increases quantity and quality of breastmilk for nursing mothers. Fennel, hops, and nettle are examples.

HEART TONIC: supports emotions of the heart and eases sadness and grief. Also can support the heart muscle and help maintain a healthy heart. Rose, hibiscus, motherwort, and holy basil are heart tonics.

INFUSION: a process of brewing herbs in water to extract their properties. In an infusion, you brew the softer parts of a plant, such as the flowers and leaves. Contrary to a "typical brew" in which you steep herbs eight to twelve minutes and strain, an infusion is steeped several hours and often left in the lidded pot overnight on the counter. It is then strained and drunk as a strong tea; often mild herbs taste stronger with this method, and infusions extract more minerals from plants than a simple brew.

MARC: the wet herbs left over after extracting in a liquid; can be composted.

NERVINE TONIC: supports a healthy nervous system and eases anxiety and stress. Catnip, lavender, rose, chamomile, borage, hibiscus, holy basil, motherwort, turmeric, and St. John's wort, among others, are nervine tonics.

OXYMEL: a medicinal blend of sweet and sour—for instance, herb-infused vinegar with honey or herb-infused lemon juice with sugar. Strong-tasting herbs such as garlic are often made into oxymels.

SEDATIVE: promotes sleep, helpful for insomnia and poor sleep. Catnip and lavender are mild sedatives; valerian and hops are stronger.

VULNERARY: helps to heal wounds on the skin, easing inflammation and repairing tissue. Calendula, lavender, yarrow, plantain, and many more are vulnerary.

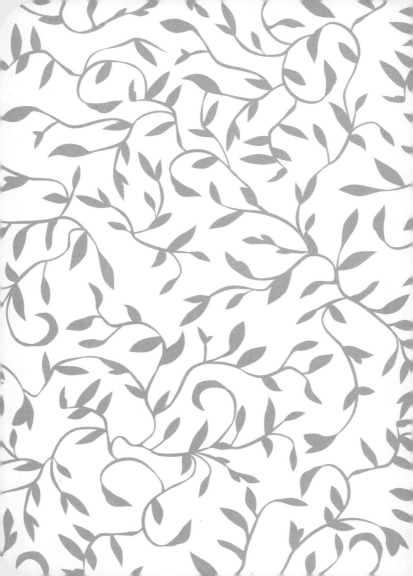